AF616712

Pediatric Endoscopy

The Principles and Practice of the Pediatric Surgical Specialties

Edited by Stephen L. Gans, M.D.
Clinical Professor of Surgery
School of Medicine
University of California, Los Angeles
Attending in Surgery
Children's Hospital of Los Angeles
and Cedars-Sinai Medical Center
Los Angeles, California

This is the first book in the series.

Pediatric Endoscopy

Edited by

Stephen L. Gans, M.D.

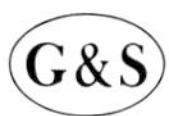

Grune & Stratton

A Subsidiary of Harcourt Brace Jovanovich, Publishers
New York London
Paris San Diego San Francisco São Paulo
Sydney Tokyo Toronto

Figure 1. *View of the postnasal space of a 3-year-old child showing a posterior congenital choanal atresia on the right side. On the left side, the posterior ends of the inferior turbinate and the middle turbinate can be seen. A small amount of adenoid tissue is on the roof of the nasopharynx. (Benjamin)*

Figure 2. *The normal larynx of an infant. The supraglottic tissues include the prominent epiglottis, the aryepiglottic folds, and the arytenoids. Anterior to the glossoepiglottic folds are the valleculae. The piriform fossae are seen on each side with the postcricoid region between them. The vocal cords and the glottic aperture are clearly visible. (Benjamin)*

Figure 3. *A large mass of papillomata that almost fills the glottic aperture. It is growing from the right hemilarynx of a 4-year-old child. (Benjamin)*

Figure 4. *Bilateral vocal nodules in a 5-year-old child. They are present on the medial edge of the anterior third of the vocal cords, but the anterior commissure is clear. It is usual to see minimal edema of the vocal cords themselves. (Benjamin)*

Figure 5. *A moderate-sized congenital glottic web in an infant. This is a thin membranous web. (Benjamin)*

Figure 6. *View showing the effects of an endotracheal tube that has been in situ in the larynx of an infant for 5 days. Intubation trauma in the form of ulceration of the edge of the vocal cords and in the posterior commissure can be clearly seen. (Benjamin)*

Figure 7. *Acute laryngotracheobronchitis, or "croup," in an infant. There are minimal inflammation and edema of the vocal cords, but the subglottic space is grossly swollen and edematous with serious airway obstruction necessitating tracheotomy. (Benjamin)*

Figure 8. *View showing the subcarina between the continuation of the left main bronchus (right side of figure) and the lingula (left side). On the far left is the opening of the apical segment of the left lower lobe. (Benjamin)*

Figure 9. *View at midtrachea in a newborn with esophageal atresia and tracheo-esophageal fistula. The fistulous opening on the posterior wall of the trachea is clearly shown. (Benjamin)*

Figure 10. *Total compression of the opening of the left main bronchus by a ballooned pulmonary artery arising from pulmonary hypertension. (Benjamin)*

Figure 11. *Large varices at the lower end of the esophagus in a child with portal hypertension. (Benjamin)*

Figure 12. *A coin impacted in the upper end of the esophagus for several days. Some ulceration and a little slough can be seen where the coin has impacted. (Benjamin)*

Figure 13. *Dilatation of esophageal stenosis with a Fogarty balloon catheter (from 16-mm movie film strip). (Gans)*

Figure 14. *The metallic guide wire of an Eder-Puestow dilator passing through a stricture of the esophagus (from flexible endoscope). (Cadranel)*

Figure 15. *Injection of corticosteroids at the proximal edge of an esophageal stricture (flexible endoscope). (Cadranel)*

Figure 16. *An esophagus 24 hours after ingestion of a caustic solution (16-mm movie film strip). (Gans)*

Figure 17. *The same esophagus as in Figure 16, 2 weeks later (16-mm movie film strip). (Gans)*

Figure 18. *Acute esophagitis in a 2-day-old-infant due to reflux associated with a hiatus hernia. The patient suffered severe hemorrhage from this ulcerated area (16-mm movie film strip). (Gans)*

Figure 19. *Chronic esophagitis in a teenager with reflux (flexible endoscope). (Cadranel)*

Figure 20. *Retrovision of the cardial region seen from the gastric cavity with the flexible gastroscope in the U-turn position. Note the large hiatus hernia surrounding the shaft of the fiberscope. (Cadranel)*

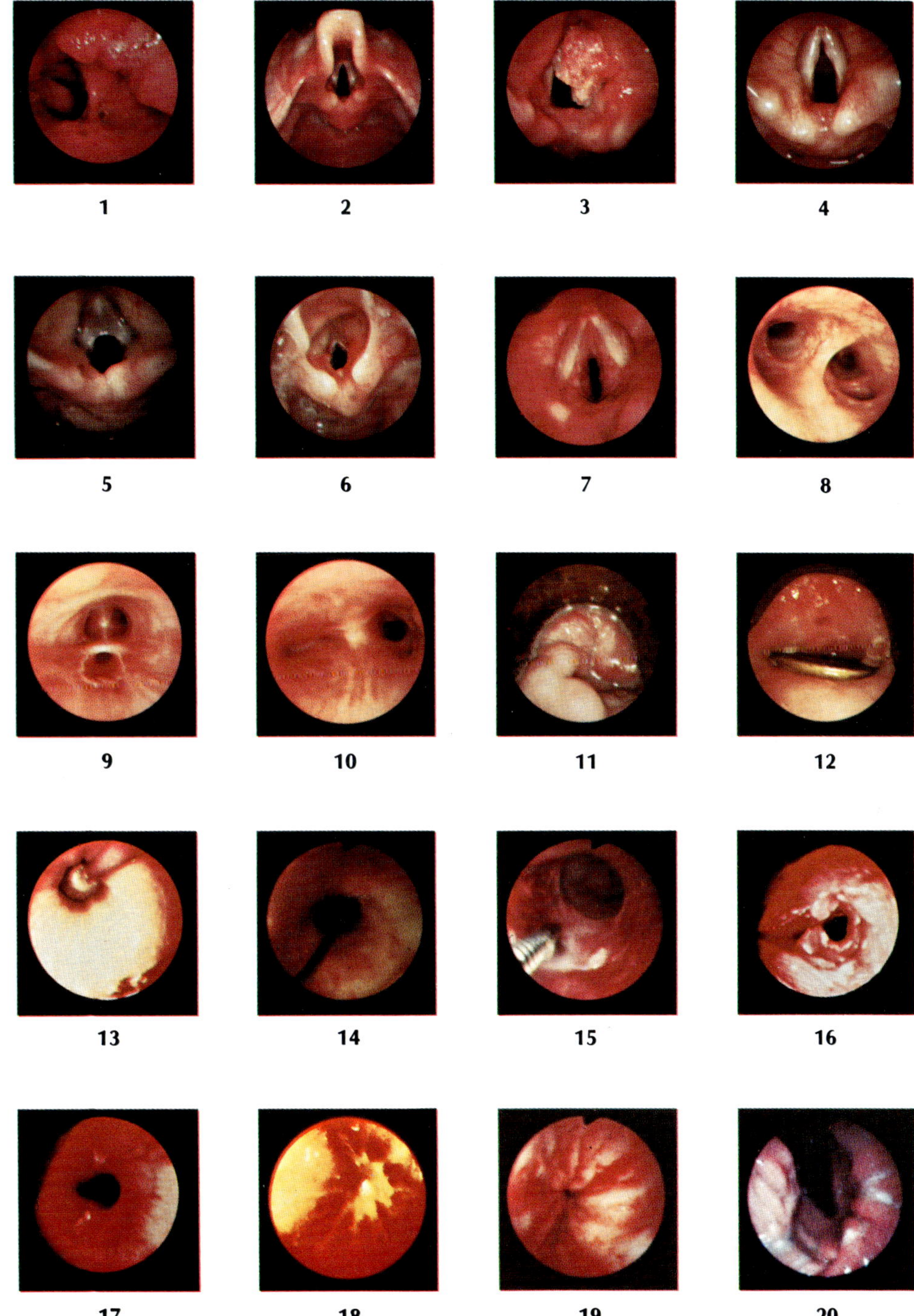

1 2 3 4

5 6 7 8

9 10 11 12

13 14 15 16

17 18 19 20

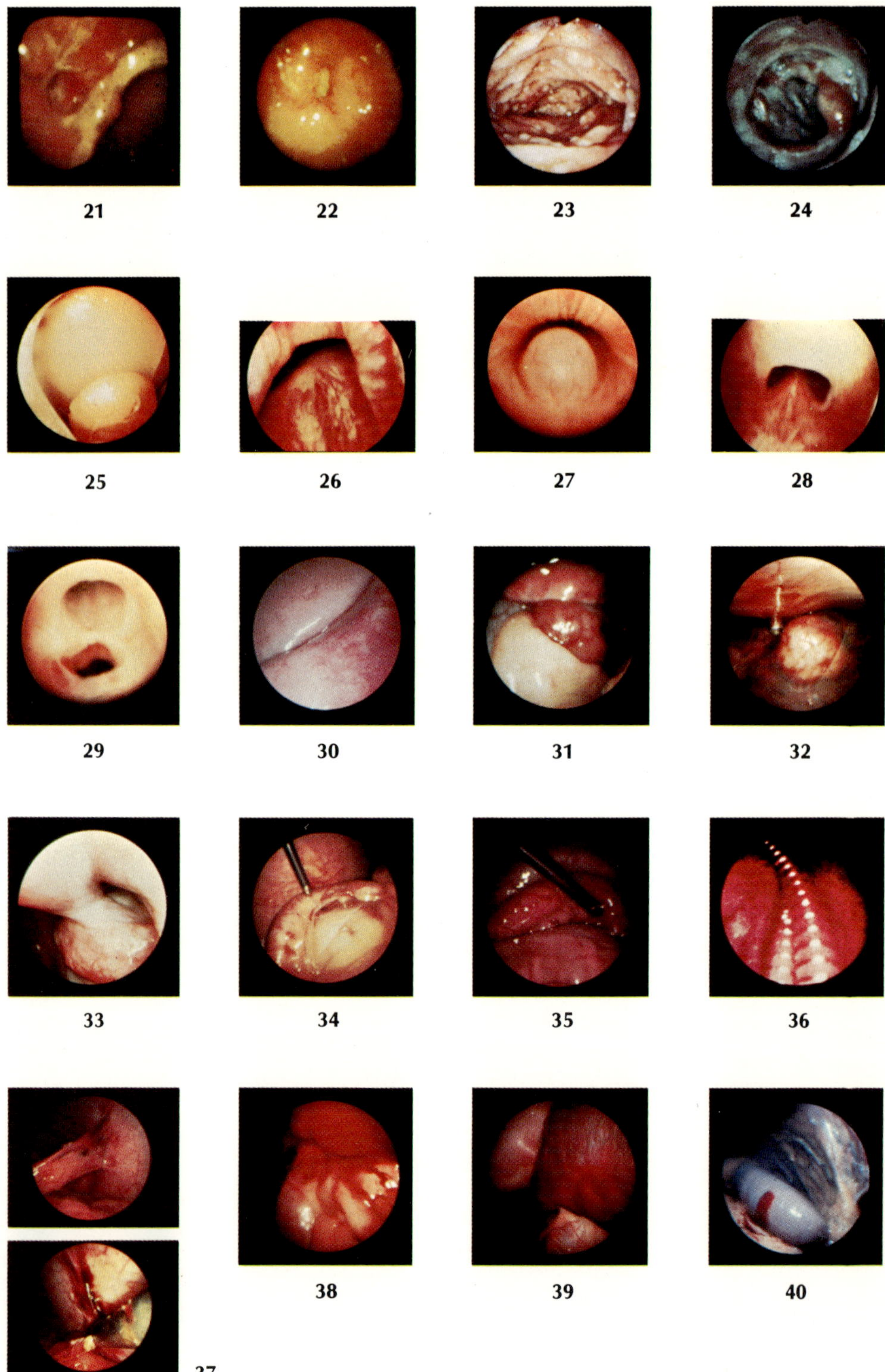
21 22 23 24
25 26 27 28
29 30 31 32
33 34 35 36
37 38 39 40

Figure 21. *A punched-out gastric ulcer in a 1-year-old child with hematemesis. An older sibling had peptic ulcer disease (flexible endoscope). (Gans)*

Figure 22. *A gastric ulcer in a child with abdominal pain (flexible endoscope). (Cadranel)*

Figure 23. *Follicular hyperplasia of the duodenum in a child (flexible endoscope). (Cadranel)*

Figure 24. *Jejunitis following gastrectomy in a teenager (flexible endoscope). (Cadranel)*

Figure 25. *A polyp in the transverse colon of a 4-year-old child (flexible endoscope). (Gans)*

Figure 26. *A large ureterocele almost completely occluding the bladder neck opening in a male. (Hendren)*

Figure 27. *A Cowper's duct cyst on the floor of the urethra in an 8-year-old boy. (Hendren)*

Figure 28. *Type 1 urethral valves. Note the two sail-like leaflets that arise from the crista and converge at 12 o'clock to form a diaphragm. (Hendren)*

Figure 29. *View of the vagina (lower opening) entering the urethra adjacent to the external urethral sphincter in a patient with mixed gonadal dysgenesis. (Hendren)*

Figure 30. *Thoracoscopic view of the minor fissure of the patient described on page 142. The pulmonary parenchyma has a pale and edematous appearance characteristic of* Pneumocystis carinii *pneumonia. The edge of the lung in the fissures appears blunted. (Rodgers)*

Figure 31. *View of the right hilum showing a large right hilar lymph node. Biopsy revealed the presence of Hodgkins disease. (Rodgers)*

Figure 32. *Hepatocarcinoma in an 8-year-old child. The tumor was well localized, and the rest of the liver and peritoneal surfaces showed no metastases. (Gans)*

Figure 33. *A twisted ovarian cyst that caused pain in a 4-year-old child. (Gans)*

Figure 34. *A normal appendix. (Leape)*

Figure 35. *Acute suppurative appendicitis. (Leape)*

Figure 36. *A segment of Raimondi tube that has broken off from a ventriculoperitoneal shunt and is lying in the pelvis (16-mm movie film strip). (Gans)*

Figure 37. *Top: an omental adhesion to the parietal peritoneum. Bottom: the adhesion divided at laparoscopy. (Leape)*

Figure 38. *A severely bleeding spleen seen at bedside laparoscopy in the emergency room. (Austin)*

Figure 39. *At laparoscopy, 350 ml of blood were aspirated from the peritoneal cavity. View now shows blood clotting on the surface of the spleen and very little bleeding. (Austin)*

Figure 40. *Laparoscopy demonstrating a lacerated spleen with a clot filling the laceration and no active bleeding. (Gans)*

Grune & Stratton, Inc.
111 Fifth Avenue
New York, New York 10003

Distributed in the United Kingdom by
Academic Press Inc. (London) Ltd.
24/28 Oval Road, London NW 1

Library of Congress Catalog Number 83-48118
International Standard Book Number 0-8089-1547-9

Printed in the United States of America

To my father,
whose brilliant and thoughtful concept of our world
was dimmed only by his impaired eyesight,
and to my mother, who was his eyes, his strength,
and a reflection of his character

Contents

Preface

A new era in pediatric endoscopy began in the 1970s due to the technical and optical achievements described in the first chapter of this book. Because of the advanced state of his knowledge of these inventions and his creative foresight in recognizing their advantages, Dr. George Berci entered the endoscopic arena armed only with sets of new drawings to support his prior experience. Encouraged and instructed by Dr. Berci, I undertook the investigation of the pediatric aspect of this field, and through the generous financial support of Mr. and Mrs. Samuel Schulman, the prototype pediatric instruments were brought from Germany in 1969 for clinical trial and use. The first bronchoscopy and esophagoscopy in a neonate, using Hopkins telescopes and fiberoptic lighting, were performed by us at the Cedars of Lebanon Hospital in Los Angeles in January 1970. Color movies were made of this procedure. The first views were indescribably thrilling. In the next few months equally exciting moments were provided by the use of these new instruments in peritoneoscopy (now referred to as laparoscopy) and in urethrocystoscopy.

In August 1970 Dr. C. Everett Koop invited me to Philadelphia to describe our early experiences at an open forum, and as a result of this he asked me to prepare a supplement for the *Journal of Pediatric Surgery* that would describe all of the instruments available at that time and detail their use. The supplement was published in April 1971 and was a precursor or "early edition" of this book.[1]

Visits with Mr. Karl Storz at his plant in Germany provided an opportunity to work out problems with and obtain improvements over the original prototype instruments. Mr. Storz was always most accommodating and understanding; he was also a perfectionist about providing optimum results.

Knowing of my interest in endoscopy, the Olympus Company of Japan invited me to visit their engineers in Tokyo in 1972 to help develop a pediatric flexible gastrointestinal endoscope. A few months later they delivered to me a prototype instrument that became their first-generation pediatric gastrointestinal fiberscope. We had previously used the flexible adult bronchoscope for examination of the stomach and duodenum in infants, but this new flexible scope gave us an opportunity to evaluate better its usefulness at both ends of the gastrointestinal tract. With very little help

[1] Gans SL, Berci G: Advances in endoscopy of infants and children. J Pediatr Surg 6:199–234, 1971

from the literature, and none from other centers, we developed methods, safeguards, indications, and contraindications for the flexible endoscope and presented this work at the meeting of the American Academy of Pediatrics, Surgical Section, in San Francisco on October 19, 1974. Our paper—one of the first on the subject—was published in 1975.[2] New generations of flexible endoscopes made by several manufacturers are now available and are described in appropriate chapters.

This book is by no means a compendium of all conditions in which endoscopy is involved. Rather it is intended to explain the advances that have so radically changed and broadened the field of pediatric endoscopy. Included is a chapter on the improvements now available in teaching and photodocumentation. The remaining chapters outline indications for specific endoscopic examinations, explain in detail how to do them, list contraindications, and mention possible complications and how to avoid them.

The authors were selected because they are acknowledged authorities in the area of their contributions. They have been permitted enough latitude to express themselves so that each chapter has its own flavor. I would like to thank them for giving of their knowledge and experience and for their cooperation and patience in the production of this book.

Many thanks are also due to the staff of Grune & Stratton for the countless ways in which they provided assistance when needed.

Finally, much gratitude is due to George Berci, who provided the thought, stimulation, encouragement, and instruction that involved me so deeply in the field of pediatric endoscopy; as a result, I have been able to share this improved "view" and give an added dimension to the better care of infants and children.

---

[2] Gans SL, Ament M, Christie DL, et al: Pediatric endoscopy with flexible fiberscopes. J Pediatr Surg 10:375–380, 1975

Contributors

Edward Austin, M.D., Attending in Surgery, Cedars-Sinai Medical Center; Chief, Division of General Surgery, Century City Hospital, Los Angeles, California

Bruce Benjamin, O.B.E., M.B., B.S., D.L.O., F.R.A.C.S., Lecturer in Diseases of the Ear, Nose, and Throat, Sydney University; Ear, Nose, and Throat Surgeon, Royal Alexandra Hospital for Children, Sydney, Australia

George Berci, M.D., F.A.C.S., Associate Director of Surgery, Cedars-Sinai Medical Center; Associate Clinical Professor of Surgery, School of Medicine, University of California, Los Angeles, Los Angeles, California

Samy Cadranel, M.D., Head, Pediatric Gastroenterology Unit, Hospital Saint-Pierre, University of Brussels, Brussels, Belgium

Stephen L. Gans, M.D., Clinical Professor of Surgery, School of Medicine, University of California, Los Angeles; Attending in Surgery, Children's Hospital of Los Angeles and Cedars-Sinai Medical Center, Los Angeles, California

W. Hardy Hendren, M.D., Professor of Surgery, Harvard Medical School; Chief of Surgery, Children's Hospital; Visiting Surgeon, Massachusetts General Hospital, Boston, Massachusetts

Hans Huchzermeyer, M.D., Professor of Medicine, Division of Gastroenterology and Hepatology, Department of Medicine, Hannover Medical School, Hannover, West Germany

Lucian L. Leape, M.D., Professor of Surgery, School of Medicine, Tufts University; Chief of Pediatric Surgery, New England Medical Center Hospital, Boston, Massachusetts

Pierre Rodesch, M.D., Chef de Clinique Adjoint, Pediatric Gastroenterology Unit, Hospital Saint-Pierre, University of Brussels, Brussels, Belgium

Bradley M. Rodgers, M.D., Professor of Surgery and Pediatrics, School of Medicine, University of Virginia; Chief, Division of Pediatric Surgery, University of Virginia Hospital, Charlottesville, Virginia

Urs G. Stauffer, M.D., Vice-Director of Pediatric Surgery, University Children's Hospital; Professor of Pediatric Surgery, Faculty of Medicine, University of Zurich, Zurich, Switzerland

James L. Talbert, M.D., Professor and Chief, Division of Pediatric Surgery, University of Florida, Gainesville, Florida

John K. Vries, M.D., Chief, Pediatric Neurosurgery and Associate Professor of Neurological Surgery, University of Pittsburgh, Pittsburgh, Pennsylvania

Christopher B. Williams, B.M., F.R.C.P., Consultant Physician, St. Mark's Hospital for Diseases of Rectum and Colon and St. Bartholomew's Hospital; Honorary Consultant Physician, Hospital for Sick Children and Queen Elizabeth Hospital for Children, London, England

Principles of Optics and Illumination

CHAPTER 1

Stephen L. Gans

Somewhat more than a century of experimentation and development passed before pediatric endoscopy emerged from the "dark ages." The medical profession had long been aware of the advantage and need of direct inspection and manipulative procedures inside hollow organs or cavities. Bozzini considered the possibility of endoscopic examination in 1806. He devised a wax candle with a mirror reflector for illumination, but it is doubtful that he saw further than the cricopharyngeal sphincter. The real beginning of endoscopy occurred in the 1860s with the work of Desormeaux and Kussmaul.[1]

Desormeaux (in Paris) designed an open tube endoscope for use in the urethra and bladder. For illumination he used the light of a small flame reflected through a lens for condensation. Realizing the possibilities of this instrument, Kussmaul (in Freiburg) sent one of his assistants to visit Desormeaux to learn about that endoscope and its possibilities for esophagoscopy. Hitherto it had been assumed that a tube had to be fitted with some form of mirror, prism, or reflector to overcome the angle made by the horizontal axis of the mouth and the vertical axis of the pharynx and esophagus.

The solution to this problem fortuitously appeared at an inn in Freiburg, called the Wolfschlucht, much frequented by students and clinical assistants at the medical school nearby. Here, a professional sword swallower performed his act, and one of the assistants, fascinated by the feat, persuaded the sword swallower to visit the clinic for observation by Kussmaul. Noting that the previously mentioned angle could be overcome by proper positioning of the head and neck, Kussmaul had a local instrument maker fashion tubes of the Desormeaux type, and introduced them into the gullet of his willing subject. For illumination he used the reflected light of a gasogen (a mixture of alcohol and turpentine) lamp. The view was hindered by poor lighting, fluid collection, and reflux, but it was a notable accomplishment and the start of a new art. In this same decade examinations were also described by Bevan, Waldenburg, and Stoerk with individually created instruments.[1]

Although many others followed this lead, the next significant development in endoscopy was the introduction of electric lighting and of the miniature Edison lamp. Now the classical endoscope became an open tube with a proximal or distal electric light source (Figure 1-1A). For a variety of examinations and procedures this arrangement has been used for many years, and it is still the method of choice in some clinics. Although quite acceptable for adults, when reduced in size for pediatric use the field of view becomes very small and the image dim and less than satisfactory. If one uses a tube with a small diameter, such as the one used for infant bronchoscopy, for example, with an inside diameter of 3.0 mm and a 200-mm length, the visual field is determined by the diameter of the small tube—3.0 mm at one end is 3.0 mm at the other end (Figure 1-1A). The addition of a magnifying loupe at the proximal end does not change the size of the visual field. Because of the tiny view and the long focal distance through the tube, only a very small part of the organ is visible and, for this reason, orientation is difficult and illumination is inadequate.

The next advance was a logical one: the use of a telescope that would transmit an image from a deep hole to the examiner's eye when properly illuminated. In 1879 Nitze developed such a lens system and introduced the first cystoscope.[2] This system became a standard over the years. Although there were many modifications and improvements, the basic principle of the telescope remained the same: small lenses placed at intervals with air space between them (Figure 1-1B). Although the viewing angle was increased, it remained small; but a greater drawback was the enormous light absorption by the lens system. Again, this telescope is reasonably satisfactory for adults, but when the diameter is decreased for pediatric use the light absorption becomes even more significant and the image is quite dim as compared with that obtainable in adults.

To this point, then, the limiting factor in pediatric endoscopy had always been the size of the instrument. With the open tube bronchoscopes and esophagoscopes, and with the conventional telescopes used in urethrocystoscopy and laparoscopy, the field of view is too small and too dim, making orientation difficult and the image less than satisfactory. As a result, a large number of endoscopic procedures in infants and children have been unduly prolonged, repeated, or even abandoned, even in skillful and experienced hands. In addition, teaching and learning of this art has been difficult and lengthy.

We owe much to the pioneers with their makeshift lamps, who, literally groping in the dark, helped to pave the way to more modern techniques. Furthermore, we can have nothing but awe and admiration for those in the pediatric field who have practiced this art with more modern but still inadequate tools, who were sometimes able to see so much under such difficult circumstances.

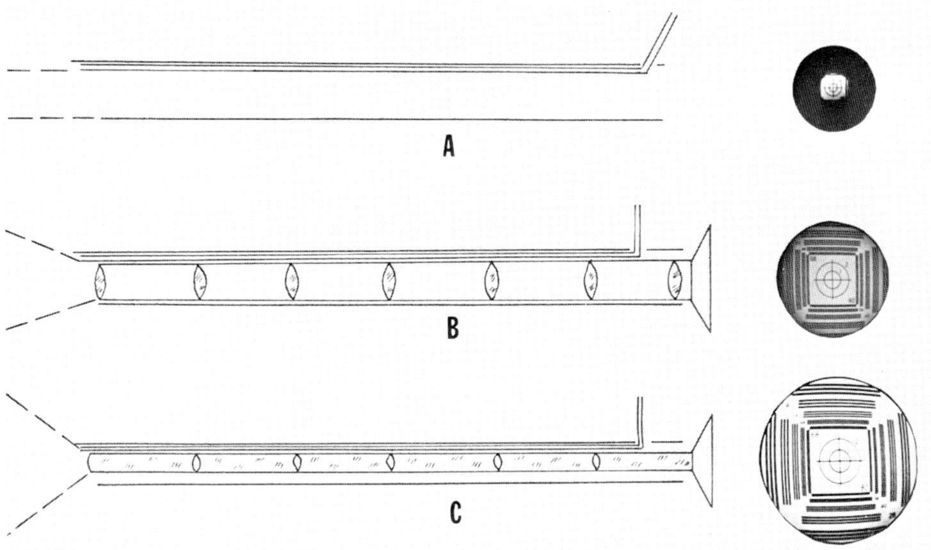

Figure 1-1. *Progressive improvements in endoscopic instrumentation. (A) Conventional open tube endoscope used for bronchoscopy and esophagoscopy. Diameter measures 3 mm and lumen is partially occluded by light carrier. Size of field of view (right) is same as both ends, even if magnifying loupe is used. (B) Endoscope of same size but with conventional telescope. Small lenses (shaded) are separated by large air spaces. Field of view (right) is somewhat increased but much light is lost in transmission, making image relatively dim. (C) Endoscope of same size but with the Hopkins rod lens telescope, in which long rod lenses (shaded) are separated by short air spaces. Image transmission is greatly increased and field of view is expanded. Fiberoptic filaments along lens system carry strong symmetric light beam directly to object. Innermost circle in field of view (right) represents area 2 mm in diameter. There is also room between sheath and telescope for ventilation (in bronchoscopy) and for passage of instruments. (From Gans SL, Berci G: Inside tracheoesophageal fistula: New endoscopic approaches. J Pediatr Surg 8:205, 1973. With permission.)*

Two technical advances have done much to improve this situation[3]:

1. The *invention by Hopkins of a rod lens optical system* for telescopes,[4] making possible miniature *rigid* endoscopic instruments that provide clear, magnified, wide-angle images and capabilities never before possible.
2. The *development of fiberoptic principles,* resulting in both brilliant and dependable illumination as well as the achievement of an image through a flexible endoscope.

Let us examine these advances in greater detail.

Advanced Optical Systems

The Hopkins rod lens system reverses the traditional arrangement of lenses in a telescope. Instead of using small lenses with intervening air spaces, Hopkins used glass rods in place of the air spaces, and small air spaces in place of the usual small lenses (Figure 1-1C). The ends of the glass rods were shaped in the form of a lens.

With this ingenious optical system, the *viewing angle is significantly larger*, there is *increased light transmission* and exceedingly *good resolution*, and *miniaturization* is feasible with exceptional performance.

Viewing angle. The viewing angle is two to three times larger than in conventional systems, depending on the object distance. A much greater part of the organ can thus be seen in a single viewing field. This makes orientation much easier. The view is more realistic and the examination can be accomplished faster. If any questionable areas are seen, the scope is brought closer and the object image enlarged, allowing more detailed inspection.

Light transmission. As previously mentioned, the degree of light absorption through a small telescope is very high, and this limits the efficiency of the conventional systems. The Hopkins system has the distinct advantage, by comparison, of a significant increase in light transmission with a much brighter image.

Optical resolution. Optical resolution is excellent, and lesions 0.5 mm in size can be detected easily from a distance of 25 mm. The physiology of vision imposes a limit on the resolution when looking through the usual infant bronchoscope, which has such a small lumen (3 mm) and a comparatively great length (200 mm). Moreover, if the object distance is 15 mm from the working end of the tube, the size of the field (object) is still no more than 3 mm. With the Hopkins telescopic system, which has identical object–objective distance, the object image is transmitted to the receptor system under significantly improved conditions. This system produces enlargement and increased brightness, the size of the object seen through the telescope being 18 mm in diameter as compared with 3 mm through the open tube.

Miniaturization. The diameter of the telescope is an important factor in determining the outside diameter of an endoscopic instrument. This is of extreme importance relative to pediatric anatomy, where the various orifices and organs are of small size, particularly in the newborn. Not only can this Hopkins lens system permit significant miniaturization, but it even leaves room in the endoscope for instrumental passage and use in front of the telescope (Figures 1-1C, 1-2).

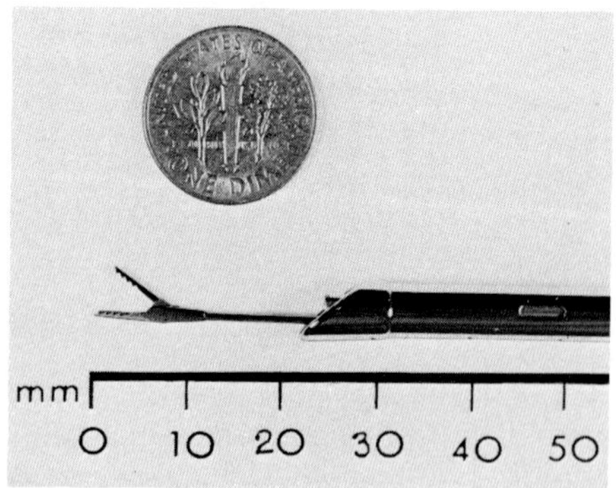

Figure 1-2. *Demonstration of a 4-mm esophagoscope with the end of the telescope just inside the lip. A grasping forceps has been passed through the instrument channel of the endoscope, and its operation is in direct view of the telescope.*

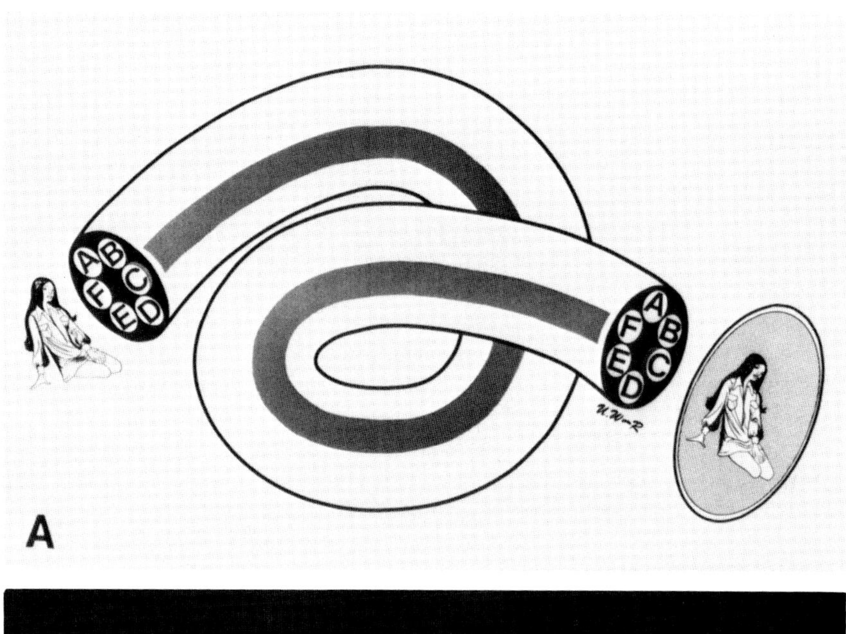

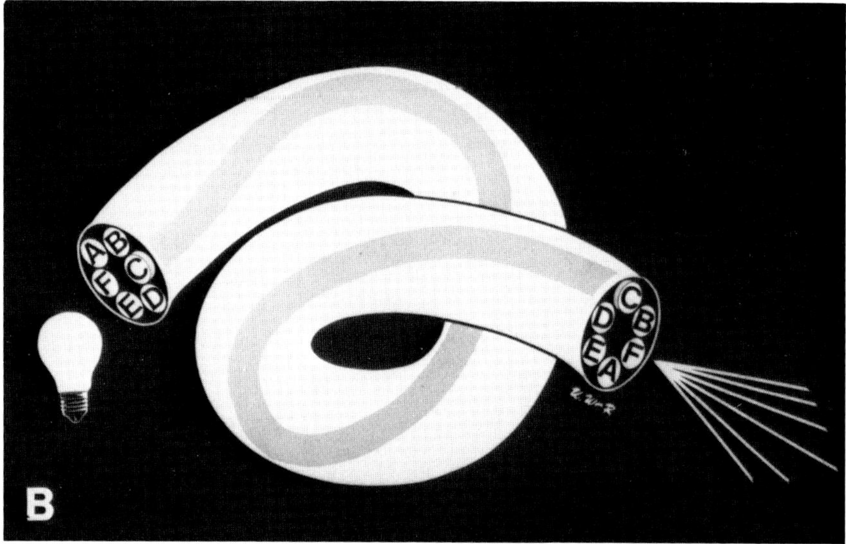

Figure 1-3. *(A) Coherent bundle. The glass fibers are in the same relationship to each other at both ends and thus transmit an image. (B) Incoherent bundle. Glass fibers are haphazardly arranged and will transmit light only. (From Gans SL, Ament M, Christie DL, et al: Pediatric endoscopy with flexible fiberscopes. J Pediatr Surg 10:375–380, 1975. With permission.)*

Fiberoptic Principles

The conventional endoscope illuminates the field by the introduction of a light carrier down to the working end of the endoscope through a small guide tube that is incorporated into the wall of the scope. Only tiny light globes can be used; thus, there are greatly limited light output and unilateral illumination. The object seen is not uniformly illuminated, and so there are significant contrast differences on the object that can be confusing in assessing small changes. Globes tend to burn out and are easily covered with secretions or blood obscuring the view. In addition, the light carrier itself occupies 1.6 mm of the diameter and when recessed in the wall of the scope either decreases the viewing angle or increases the outside diameter, a significant factor in a bronchoscope with a 3.0-mm lumen.

The most significant forward step in obtaining improved illumination was the development of small flexible fiberglass threads for the transmission of light. In 1930 Lamm (in London) described his successful experiment in transmitting light through small individual fiber threads held together in a flexible bundle.[3] If the individual fiber threads are sorted with great care (Figure 1-3A), an image can be transmitted even when the bundle is in a bent position. This is called a *coherent bundle*. If the individual fiber threads are not assorted appropriately, each thread will not transmit its respective part of the image in position and the image will be distorted, although *light is still transmitted*. These nonassorted fiber threads are called *incoherent bundles* (Figure 1-3B); they can be attached on one end to a light source at some distance from the endoscope (for example, 6 feet).

If fiber threads are placed around a telescope and brought out in a bent position or right angle near the eyepiece in a rigid bundle (Figure 1-4A), the flexible light-transmitting cable can then be connected from the light source to the telescope, providing transmission of the beam of the remote light source into the body cavity.

Because of the smaller diameter of the Hopkins lens systems, it is now possible to place a thin layer of light-transmitting optical fiber (incoherent) bundles around the rod lenses, thereby providing even, strong, cold light illumination without occupying significant space in the endoscope itself (Figure 1-4B). Compared with separate light-carrier systems, this has an inestimable advantage. Not only is the method more practical and trouble-free, but it creates a clear, bright view sufficiently powerful even for color photography, television, and split imaging.

The development of *coherent* fiber bundles made flexible endoscopes feasible, and several models were developed and used. Again, although quite satisfactory for adults, there are serious problems involved in miniaturization of flexible fiber image-transmitting endoscopes. When the scope diameter is decreased the resolution drops considerably, because it is proportionate to the number of threads incorporated in the system. In addition, space is needed for a control mechanism for bending the tip, for suction and irrigation, and for an instrument channel (Figure 1-5). As a result, pediatric-sized instruments have neither the image quality nor capabilities of the adult size, nor the brilliant view of the rigid endoscopes with the Hopkins system. At this time, however, one must compromise on occasions when it is necessary to enter those organs where a larger size or a rigid system is not feasible.

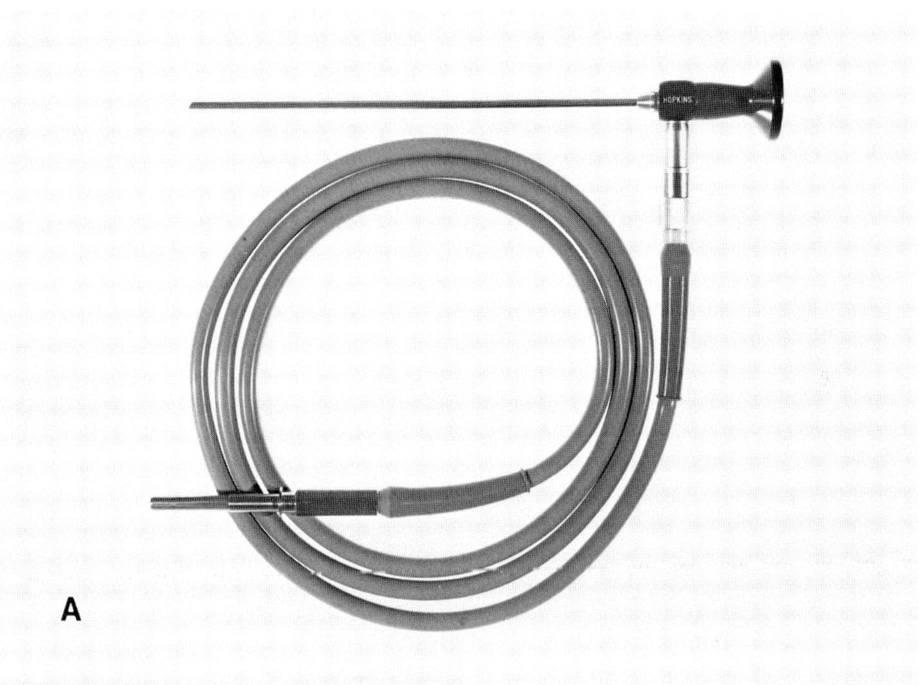

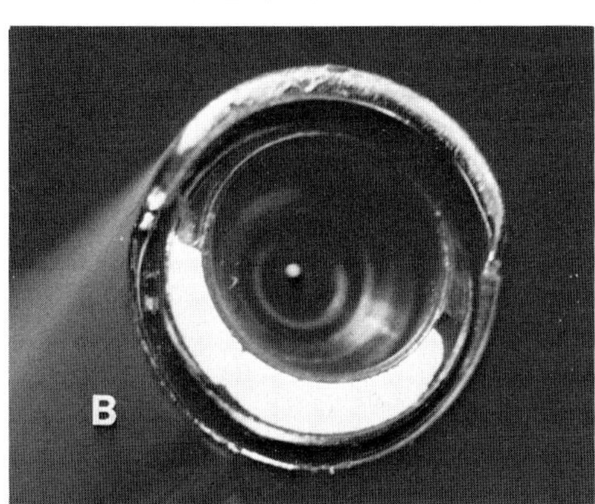

Figure 1-4. *(A) Hopkins rod lens telescope with fiber threads brought out in bent position near the eyepiece in a rigid bundle and connected to a flexible light-transmitting cable that can be plugged into a remote light source. (B) Distal end of Hopkins rod lens telescope showing illumination emanating from the fiber threads placed around the telescope lens.*

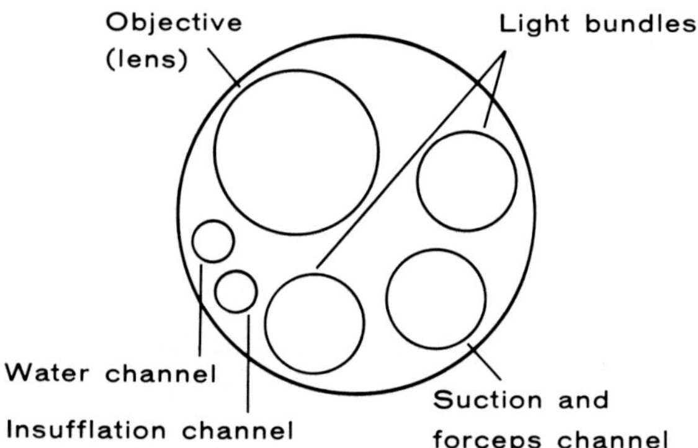

Figure 1-5. *Diagram of distal end of flexible endoscope with facilities for lighting and viewing (objective), water injection, air insufflation, suction, and passage of instruments. (From Gans SL, Ament M, Christie DL, et al: Pediatric endoscopy with flexible fiberscopes. J Pediatr Surg 10:375–380, 1975. With permission.)*

Conclusion

Although endoscopy in adults has been carried on in a relatively satisfactory manner for a long time, pediatric procedures have lagged far behind, the size of the instruments being the limiting factor. Due to significant technical advances, pediatric endoscopy came of age only in the 1970s, since which time great progress has been made and endoscopic capabilities have become more widely available and practiced. There is no doubt that endoscopists will find their skills enhanced and the benefits to their patients greatly increased by these advances. The availability of a superior instrument, however, does not necessarily make its user an expert. Knowledge and experience in this field must be combined with study and practice in order to derive the best results and greatest satisfaction.

References

1. Kelly HDB: Origins of oesophagology. Proc R Soc Med 62:781–786, 1969
2. Nitze M: Eine neue Beobachtungs und Untersuchungs Methode für Harnröhre und Harnblase. Wien Med Wochenschr 24:650, 1879
3. Gans S, Berci G: Advances in endoscopy of infants and children. J Pediatr Surg 6:199–234, 1971
4. Berci G, Kont LA: A new optical system in endoscopy with special reference to cystoscopy. Br J Urol 41:564, 1969

Teaching and Documentation of Pediatric Endoscopic Procedures

CHAPTER 2

George Berci

A permanent record of visual findings has been proven to be of utmost importance in many investigative modalities. It is the most valuable adjunct to any diagnostic procedure in which certain visual signs or appearances indicate functional or organic disorders. Diagnostic radiography provides an excellent example. The great impact in this area was the development of a method whereby x-ray films could be scrutinized under optimal viewing conditions for an unlimited time. Many minute lesions overlooked on first inspection were discovered on repeated review. In complicated cases consultation enhanced the information.

A verbal description, however accurate, cannot substitute for a print displaying actual appearance. If a patient is followed for a certain period of time, progress or regress of a lesion can be objectively assessed by analyzing x-ray films taken at time intervals. This advantage has also become important in electrocardiography, ultrasound, and many other important diagnostic examinations that provide a permanent record that can be scrutinized at leisure without overtaxing the patient.

This development is also applicable for endoscopic procedures, but the technological developments described in the preceding chapter were necessary before it could be effective in infants and children.[1] It is also true that despite the present possibilities of obtaining film records through pediatric endoscopes this art is still, from the practical point of view, in a developmental stage.

Teaching

After years of application, pediatric endoscopic areas previously unexplored were reopened, new areas were attacked, and, in general, "tunnel" or "keyhole" vision was exchanged for a panoramic view. The light transmission was sufficient to permit another dimension—simultaneous teaching. It was possible to split the image in two and to provide simultaneous observation by attaching a teaching attachment to the eyepiece.[2] This eliminated frustrating situations such as those in which the examiner saw the lesion and then asked a bystander to look at it, but during the maneuver of changing positions the introduced instrument had moved slightly, and the object was lost and the examination unnecessarily extended. Today in every pediatric endoscopic procedure where a telescope is employed a rigid teaching attachment can be coupled without interfering with the routine of the examination (Figure 2-1). The illumination is sufficient to provide a bright image to the operator and the observer. A rigid optical teaching instrument is preferred to a flexible one[2] because

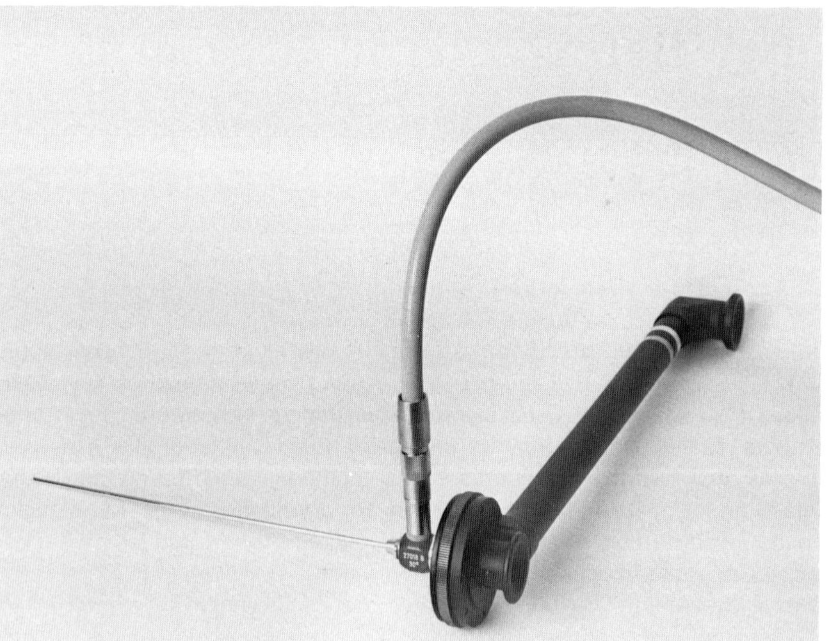

Figure 2-1. *Miniature telescope only 2.7 mm O.D. with rigid teaching attachment and flexible fiberoptic light cord. Even in this small size, the increased light transmission of the Hopkins system permits splitting of the image and provides a bright image for two simultaneous observers using a standard examining light source.*

of the significant loss of resolution in the latter. The rigid teaching attachment can be used with the flexible endoscope.

Documentation

Still Photography Through Rigid Pediatric Endoscopes

Miniature telescopes can carry only a small number of fibers because of their minute size; this is sufficient to provide enough light for examination, but it is difficult to transmit high-intensity illumination through the relatively few fibers, and the inherent packaging loss[3] further diminishes transmission (Figure 2-2). In still photography it would be ideal to use gas-discharged flash tubes and pump a high-energy discharge in a short period of time (milliseconds) through these light-carrying fibers, with a small still camera directly attached to the telescope. It is important to know that the focal length of the camera lens (50–90-mm length) plays a significant part in the size of the displayed image. If the focal length is longer the displayed image will be larger. A larger image needs significantly more light than a smaller one. Focal length, light, and image size must therefore be coordinated according to the general performance parameters, absorption factors, and film speed.[4]

The first alternative, then, is to attach a flash tube hermetically enclosed in plastic housing to the telescope and to couple an examining fiberoptic cord to the other end (Figure 2-3). Examining light is thus provided through the flash tube. A small, lightweight 35-mm camera with motor drive is attached to the eyepiece.

The advantage of this method is that it provides a maximum flash output because of the direct attachment of the flash tube to the telescope. With the camera attached (focal length: 70–90 mm) a proper photograph can be obtained. We use daylight film with a speed of ASA 200–400.

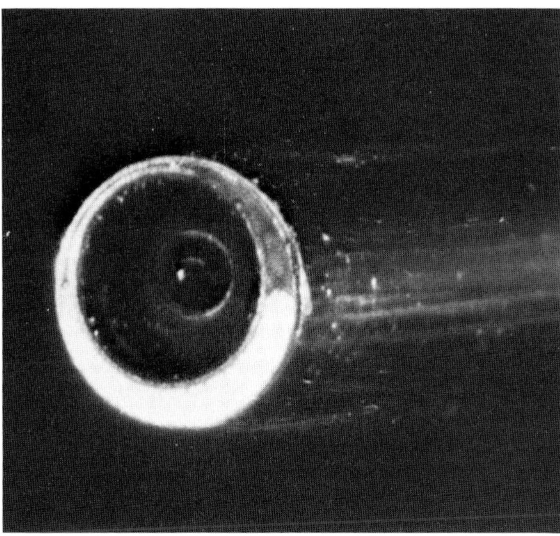

Figure 2-2. *Since the telescope* must be kept small, *only a limited number of light-conducting fibers can be used. These are more than sufficient to carry enough light for the examination, even during teaching with a split image or coupled teaching attachment (see Figure 2-1), but for photography this amount of light represents a limiting factor. This enlarged photograph displays the working tip of a pediatric telescope: objective surrounded by a minute half-moon-shaped fiber light arrangement. (Manufacturer: Karl Storz Endoscopy.)*

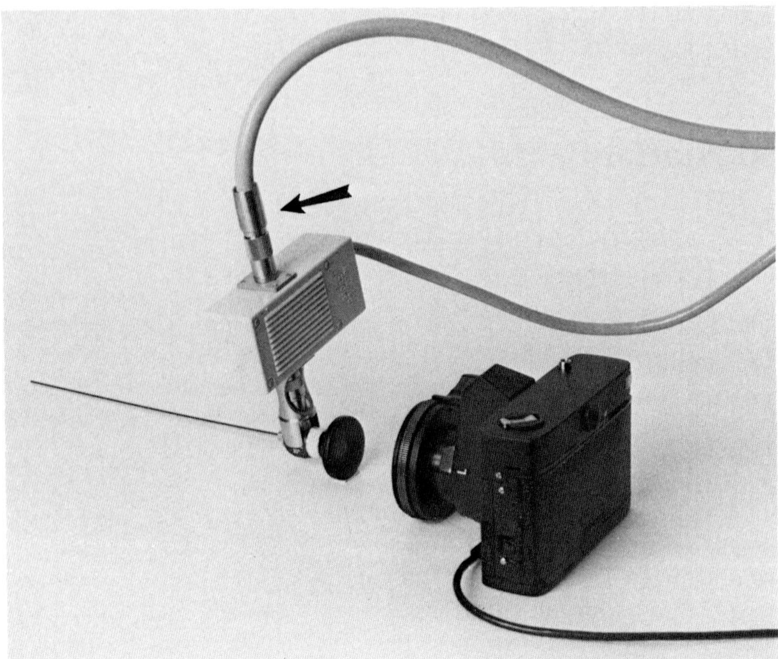

Figure 2-3. *Miniature telescope attached to one side of flash tube in a plastic housing. This flash tube assembly can be gas-sterilized if necessary. The light-carrying bundle is attached on the other side of the housing of the flash tube (arrow), providing examining light during photography.*

The disadvantages are that it is time-consuming to attach a flash tube; and for sterile procedures it must be gas-sterilized. The coupling of the camera can cause movement of the endoscope, and it can be difficult to find the proper spot through the camera viewer again. Documentation can, however, be obtained with this system, with some deviation from the examining routine.

Remote Flash System

In this case the flash generator and the tube are built together into a larger unit. The flash discharge is transmitted through a fiberoptic cable to the telescope. In the same unit, continuous examining light is also provided for the investigation (Figure 2-4). The camera is attached in the same way as in the direct flash tube system (see Figure 2-3), and the flash photograph is obtained.

The advantage of this system is that the flash tube is remotely placed. This arrangement is more convenient for the operator, and an automatic flash-meter system triggered by the attached camera can be also incorporated.

The disadvantages are that every interposed fiberoptic cable absorbs more light than a direct flash tube arrangement. Therefore, the actual output at the working end of the telescope is less; to compensate for this, a shorter photo lens (50–70 mm) is recommended.

We found that among the various modalities the following requirements should be met:

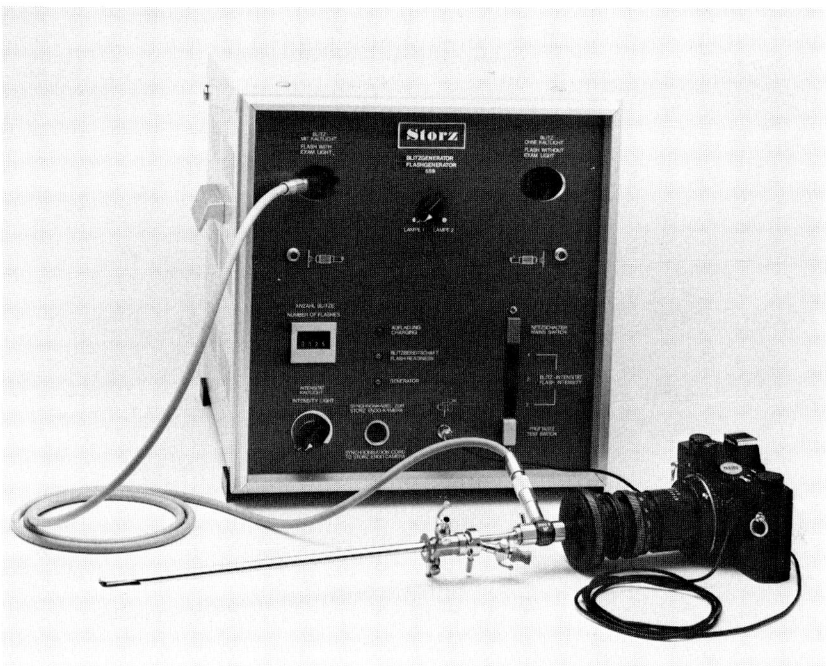

Figure 2-4. *Miniature telescope attached with fiberoptic cables to a flash unit that also contains a light source for the examination.*

1. The camera and the light unit should be kept at the remote distance from the operator.
2. The photographic techniques should not be too complicated for an endoscopist unfamiliar with photography.

To meet these needs an articulated arm was developed that consists of the Hopkins rod lens system with moving optical joints (Figure 2-5). This optical arm can easily be attached to the telescope without interfering with the actual view. The arm can be used both as a teaching attachment and for documentation because a dual beam splitter is incorporated into the eyepiece. In one position (50%/50%) the operator and the second examiner obtain the same unobstructed view, which is a great advantage for teaching. The image observed is superior to that obtained with the flexible fiberoptic teaching attachment because the image quality is maintained. The alternative position of the beam splitter gives 10 percent of the view to the operator while 90 percent is transmitted into the recording apparatus (still or movie camera or closed circuit television).

When the articulated arm is applied we employ a *high-intensity continous illuminator.* In some situations where larger telescopes in which more light-transmitting fibers are incorporated, the continuous high-intensity light source can be used in conjunction with the articulated arm, and a camera with a lens with a 50-mm focal length, shutter speed $^1/_{30}$ second, automatic film transport (winder), and film speed ASA 400. During the exposures the intensity of the light source is increased to maximum for the period of photography only. With this combination we have achieved

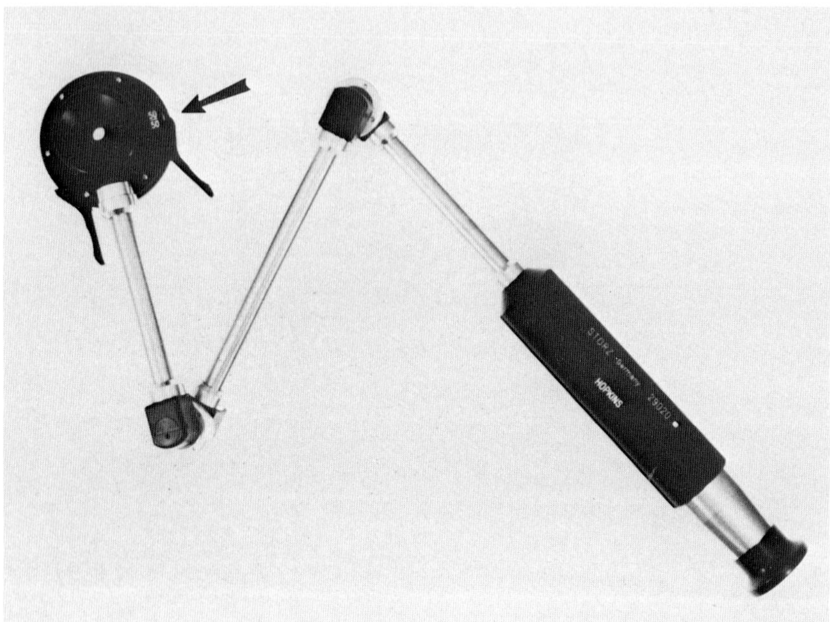

Figure 2-5. *Articulated optical arm (Hopkins rod lens system) with dual beam splitter (arrow).*

a compromise between convenience and acceptable quality of transparencies obtained within an extension of only a few minutes of our usual examining time. The camera can be released or triggered by an assistant or by using a foot switch (Figure 2-6).

Cinematography

A 16-mm movie film strip gives a "three-dimensional" view and displays movements or functional appearance. Any lightweight 16-mm movie camera with a reflex viewer directly attached to the telescope can be employed. A high-intensity light source must be used with the setting on maximum output during the filming period. The recommended focal length of the lens for cinematography is 30 mm or a maximum of 38 mm, with a wide open aperture and fixed focus. Camera speed: 16 frames/second. Film: Daylight. Speed: ASA 200. With these arrangements we have achieved excellent film strips in the newborn and infant.

Flexible Pediatric Fiberscopes

With flexible pediatric fiberscopes the light transmission or absorption parameters are less favorable than with rigid ones. One cannot expect to transmit enough light to obtain a very large image through these long (upper or lower gastrointestinal) scopes with an extended light cord of 1 mm or less in diameter. If a high-intensity light source is used, a small 16-mm *single frame* still camera, directly attached to the eyepiece of the scope, is the method of choice (Figure 2-7). The lightweight

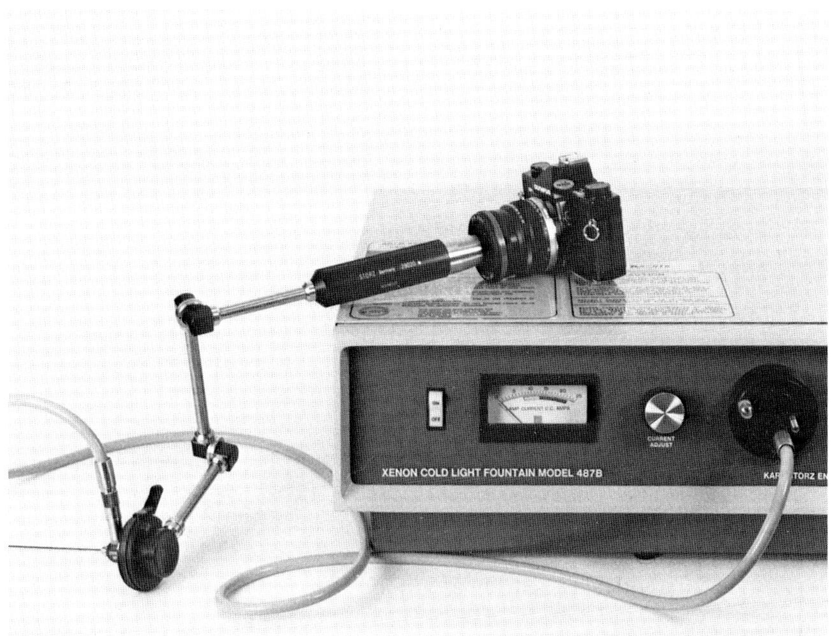

Figure 2-6. *Miniature telescope attached with a fiberoptic cable to a high-intensity (xenon) light source (Storz 487/B). The articulated optical arm is attached to the endoscope. The procedure can be performed while the examiner views through the eyepiece of the articulated arm, and the camera is exposed remotely. The same high-intensity light source can be used for cinematography or television.*

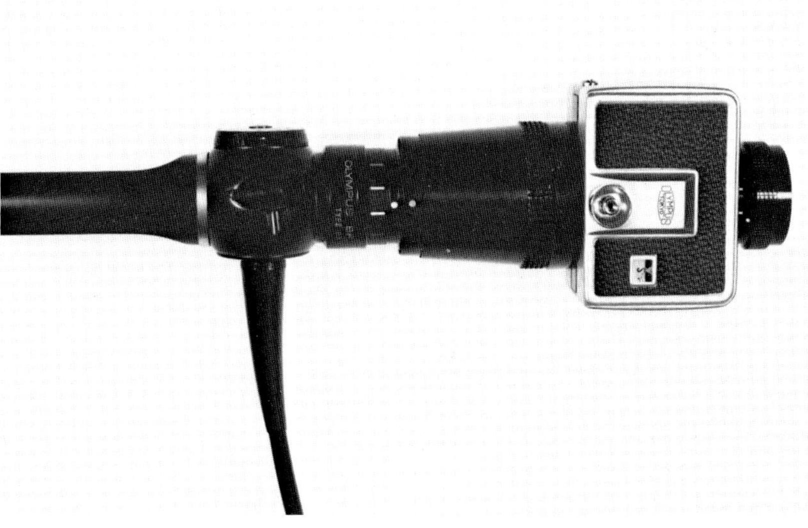

Figure 2-7. *A small 16-mm single frame camera with a reflex viewer and a motor drive (film transport) directly attached to the miniature flexible fiberscope.*

camera does not interfere with manipulation. The camera has a built-in meter determining the exposure time as well as a through the lens viewer. In cases where the distance between the object and the fiberscope tip is fairly great, exposure times of $^1/_{15}$ second or even longer are not unusual and can result in a fuzzy image.

Conclusion

The development of documentation techniques for pediatric endoscopy is still in a transitional stage. Several improvements of the present light transmission systems, light sources, or film speeds are required to simplify the methods just described. It is possible and necessary to obtain a good still photograph, or movie film strip, of an interesting pathologic or functional disorder. After the initial breakthrough in optics, pediatric endoscopy opened up many new fields of application and images never seen before were observed.

The possibility of teaching pediatric endoscopy by having the student observe the same phenomenon simultaneously is very important in training programs.

References

1. Gans S, Berci G: Advances in endoscopy in infants and children. J Pediatr Surg 6(suppl):199, 1971
2. Olson V, Berci G: Teaching attachments, in Berci G (ed): Endoscopy. New York, Appleton-Century-Crofts, 1976
3. Hopkins HH: Physics of the fiber-optic endoscope, in Berci G (ed): Endoscopy. New York, Appleton-Century-Crofts, 1976
4. Berci G, Hasler G, Helmuth JG: Permanent film records in Berci G (ed): Endoscopy. New York, Appleton-Century-Crofts, 1976

Laryngoscopy

CHAPTER 3

Bruce Benjamin

Direct examination of the larynx is the only method by which a true image of the larynx can be obtained and is the initial step in examination of the tracheobronchial tree and esophagus.

Indications and Clinical Features

The commonest indications for endoscopic assessment are to elucidate the cause of stridor, respiratory distress due to obstruction, or an abnormality of the cry or voice. Each patient must of course be evaluated individually, and babies with mild stridor or no respiratory distress may require observation only, at regular intervals. Further investigation, however, including endoscopy, is certainly indicated for severe stridor, progressive stridor, stridor associated with unusual features such as cyanotic or apneic attacks, dysphagia, aspiration, failure to thrive, or a radiologic abnormality.

Patients to be considered for endoscopy fall basically into five groups.

Neonatal airway obstruction. Congenital anomalies of the respiratory tract account for only a small percentage of persistent neonatal respiratory distress, the majority of cases being due to idiopathic respiratory distress syndrome or respiratory depression.

The obstruction may be anywhere from the nasal cavities (see Figure 1, p. v) and nasopharynx above, in the laryngopharynx, in the trachea or main bronchi below.

Serious airway obstruction in a newborn infant may be due to obvious abnormalities such as micrognathia with retroposed tongue, commonly seen in Pierre Robin syndrome; Treacher-Collins syndrome; Crouzon's disease; or macroglossia. Other causes include nasal obstruction due to bilateral posterior choanal atresia; birth trauma of the nose and nasal septum or idiopathic turbinate hypertrophy; bilateral vocal cord paralysis; congenital cyst of the pharynx or larynx; laryngeal web or stenosis; congenital subglottic stenosis; or some rare anomaly such as laryngeal atresia.

Some congenital lesions in the larynx do not present at birth, the clinical features being delayed for days or weeks; examples include laryngomalacia, congenital subglottic hemangioma, and congenital subglottic stenosis.

"Congenital laryngeal stridor." It is unfortunate that this term continues to be used by clinicians. It is not a diagnosis but an all-inclusive description.

Laryngomalacia is the commonest cause of congenital laryngeal stridor in infants. A final and confident diagnosis can be made only by direct examination of the upper respiratory tract so that the characteristic changes can be seen.

Chronic airway obstruction. Apart from conditions already discussed that may present acutely in the neonatal period (e.g., Pierre Robin syndrome), chronic, persistent, or progressive airway obstruction may be caused by an oropharyngeal mass. Cystic hygroma, ectopic thyroid tissue, or grossly enlarged tonsils and adenoids may be implicated. Other possibilities are obstruction from laryngeal papillomata, hemangioma, a laryngeal or pharyngeal cyst, and narrowing of the tracheal lumen. The stridor associated with tracheal narrowing, whether due to compression, collapse, or stenosis, is inspiratory, often with an expiratory component. A barking cough is a characteristic and prominent clinical feature of tracheal compression or collapse.

Acute inflammatory airway obstruction. The cause of airway obstruction due to acute inflammation is usually known from the clinical features assisted when necessary by x-ray findings. Acute laryngotracheitis ("croup") is by far the commonest inflammatory condition. Acute epiglottitis, although much less common, is far more dangerous and may cause death from suffocation within a few hours. In some cases a differentiation must be made from diphtheria, gross enlargement of the tonsils and adenoids with or without intercurrent infection, an unsuspected foreign body in the larynx or upper esophagus, or from one of the acute pharyngeal abscesses.

Other indications. A husky voice in an older child who previously had a normal cry raises the possibility of vocal nodules or laryngeal papillomata.

Repeated aspiration into the tracheobronchial tree in infants requires investigation for incoordinate swallowing, reflux esophagitis, bulbar palsy, H-type tracheo-esophageal fistula, or the rare cleft larynx.

A weak or absent cry, cyanotic attacks, apneic attacks, recurrent or atypical croup, and persistent or recurrent respiratory obstruction and distress may all eventually require consideration for full endoscopic examination.

Pre-Endoscopic Investigations

In older children, the larynx and pharynx can often be inspected by indirect examination with the laryngeal mirror, sometimes assisted by the use of topical anesthesia in the pharynx. This examination is not possible in infants, and clinical examination relies on evaluation of the facies, the nasal airways, the tongue, the oropharynx, and the neck together with auscultation and examination of the chest. Observation and examination over a period of hours or days may give useful information not detectable at a single examination, and where time permits such information may be extremely valuable. Other minor or major congenital abnormalities are always noted.

Although it may be possible to make a preliminary diagnosis before endoscopy, in most cases direct examination of the nasal cavities, pharynx, larynx, tracheobronchial tree, and esophagus under general anesthetic is necessary to make an exact, final, and complete diagnosis.

Radiologic studies are usually indicated and should always include an anteroposterior chest x-ray. Study of the upper airway by means of a lateral x-ray or xeroradiogram is particularly useful (Figure 3-1). A well-exposed film with the patient's head and neck in the hyperextended position has been found to provide worthwhile information, often of essential diagnostic value. Where possible this investigation should be undertaken before any patient is examined under general anesthetic, except in an emergency. In many cases the airway can be seen from the nasal cavities above, to the bifurcation of the trachea into the main bronchi below (Figure 3-2), including clear details of the soft tissues of the larynx and pharynx.

Technique of Direct Laryngoscopy

Anesthesia

General anesthesia is virtually always employed. It is very unusual indeed for patients to undergo examination without anesthesia; occasionally in sick neonates up to a few weeks of age or in those with suspected vocal cord paralysis no anesthetic will be used; but the anesthesiologist will be in attendance. Teamwork between the endoscopic surgeon and the anesthesiologist is absolutely essential.

Anesthesia should provide adequate oxygenation and carbon dioxide elimination, relaxation of the mandible and pharynx to permit gentle and leisurely examination, depression of vagal reflex activity, and in many cases retention of vocal cord movement to allow assessment of the dynamics of the larynx and pharynx.

Special problems include pre-existing hypoxia and hypercarbia and a tendency to laryngeal and bronchial spasm. Spasm or bradycardia may be produced by instrumentation of the larynx and the tracheobronchial tree. There may be a tumor, cyst, or foreign body producing an obstruction in the vicinity of the larynx so that bronchoscopy or intubation is difficult or impossible.

For premedication, atropine alone is used in babies; for older children perhaps the combination of either meperidine and atropine or papaveretum and hyoscine is

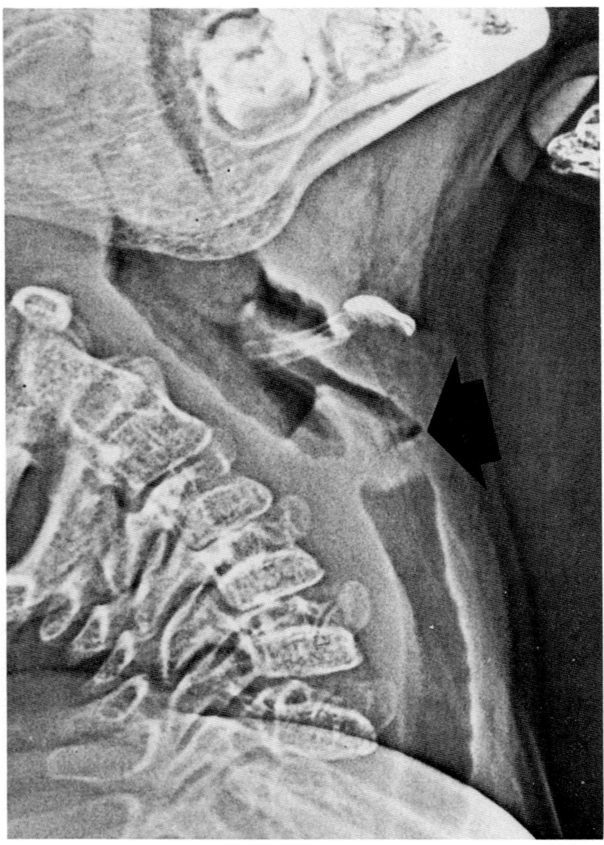

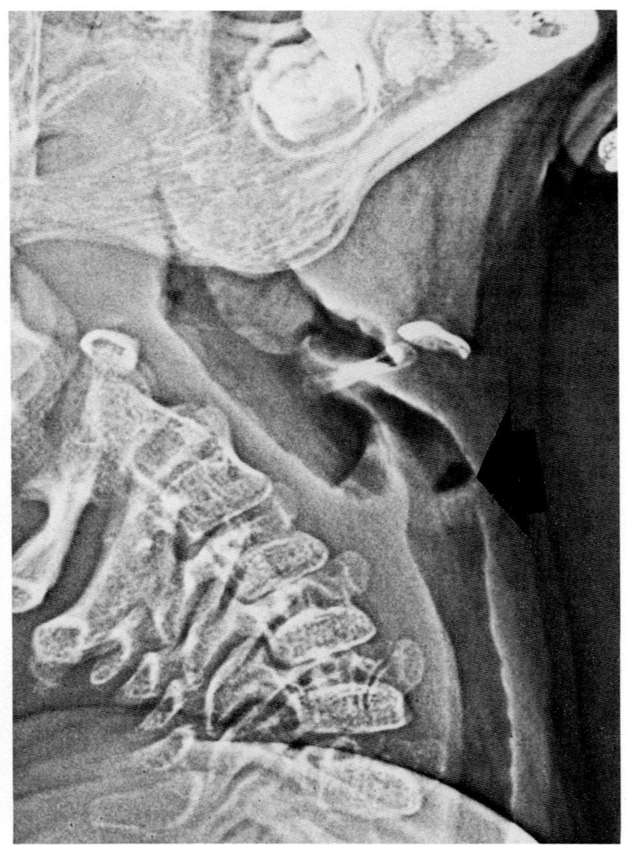

Figure 3-1. *A lateral airway xerogram is always taken with the neck in hyperextension. The ventricle of the larynx (arrow) is distinctive. Below it are the true vocal cords above the false cords and the supraglottic structures, including the epiglottis, arytenoids, aryepiglottic folds, base of the tongue, tonsils, and palate. The tracheal air column is clearly seen. Note the variation in the appearance of the glottic region, especially the true vocal cords, depending on the phase of respiration during which the film is taken.*

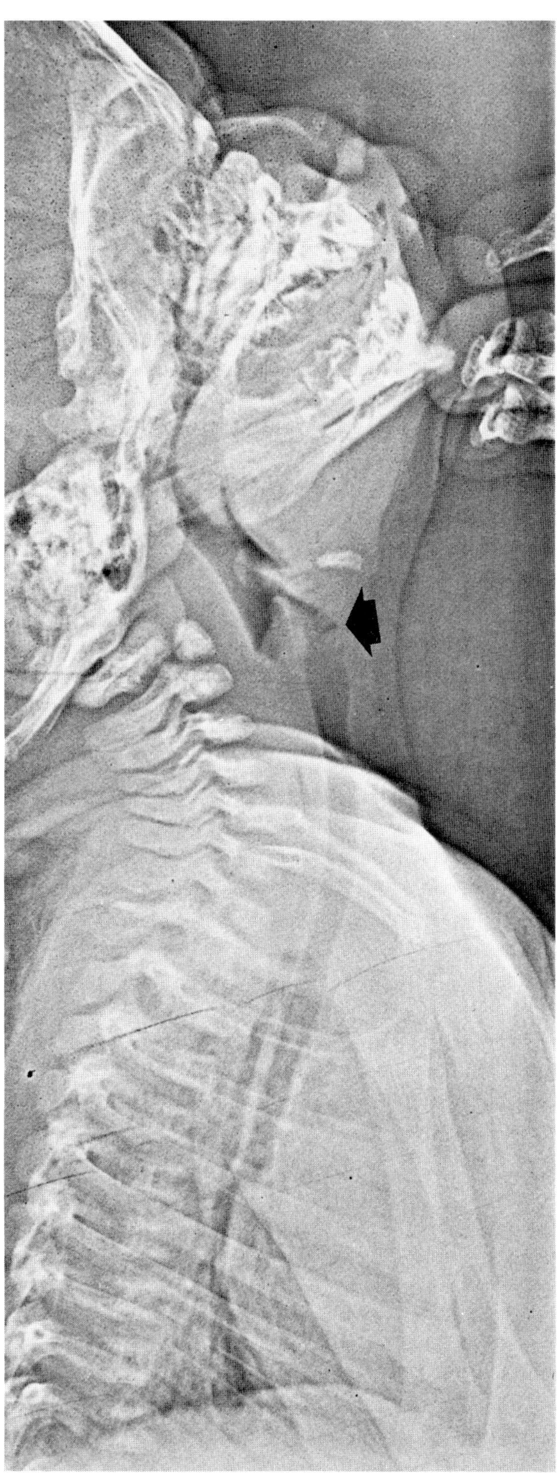

Figure 3-2. *A lateral xerogram in a normal infant showing the upper airway from the bronchi below through the trachea, larynx, pharynx, nasopharynx, and nasal airways. The arrow shows the laryngeal ventricle.*

used. The narcotic is not given in the presence of an overt degree of respiratory obstruction. If atropine has not been given by intramuscular injection it is given intravenously at or soon after induction of anesthesia. Atropine affords some protection against bradycardia and helps minimize secretions in the respiratory tract.

The most common anesthetic technique for diagnostic examination is spontaneous respiration delivered via a face mask using nitrous oxide, oxygen, and halothane; but in the case of an ill child oxygen with halothane is used. Some anesthesiologists prefer to add methoxyflurane, regarding it as a supplement to provide additional analgesia that smooths the course of the anesthesia. This spontaneous respiration technique is the method of choice in the majority of endoscopies that are diagnostic examinations. The technique is particularly suitable as it allows the opportunity for careful, unhurried observation and assessment of vocal cord movement and of the dynamic changes seen, for example, in laryngomalacia.

Topical anesthesia, up to 5 mg of lignocaine per kilogram of body weight, usually diluted to a 1 or 2 percent concentration and making a sufficient volume to handle conveniently, is sprayed on the epiglottis, larynx, and trachea to minimize unwanted reflex activity. We regard this combination of general and local anesthesia as most important. Topic analgesia has virtually abolished laryngeal spasm during endoscopy. However a venepuncture is always performed when using this technique and a muscle relaxant is always ready to be given if required.

Equipment

The laryngoscopes of Jackson with distal lighting and Negus with proximal lighting using small electric bulbs have been employed for many years, modified in size and shape for pediatric use. The development of the cold-light fountain with quartz iodine and later xenon illumination, together with flexible fiberoptic cables, now allow brilliant, cold, white light to be used for either proximal or distal illumination with added safety. A built-in second lamp in the light fountain is ready for instant use should the first one fail.

Illumination by an electronic flash generator or by a xenon light source allows endoscopic photography, still, cine, and television, to be performed as part of the routine evaluation.

We use the Storz equipment and have found it satisfactory in design, function, and safety. The light source can be used with twin flexible fiberoptic cables so that a laryngoscope and a bronchoscope are available for simultaneous use. This latter facility is especially desirable when managing a patient with an already compromised airway, as the laryngoscope may be necessary to ensure swift entry of the bronchoscope into the trachea for immediate ventilation and resuscitation. There is a range of small, proximal, prismatic light deflectors and fiberoptic light carriers to suit the particular endoscope being used. They are connected by a flexible fiberoptic cable to the light source.

Several sizes and types of Storz pediatric laryngoscopes, 8.5 cm, 9.5 cm, and 11.0 cm, are available depending on the age and size of the child. The Storz Holinger anterior commissure infant laryngoscope is a most useful instrument, not only for viewing the anterior commissure but for a larynx that is difficult to visualize with the standard laryngoscopes.

The complete range of Storz Doesel-Huzly rigid bronchoscopes includes the

2.5-mm, 3.0-mm, 3.5-mm, 4.0-mm, 5.0-mm, and the 6.0-mm instruments of varying lengths—all available with adaptations to allow ventilation. The size marked on the bronchoscope refers to the inside diameter of the lumen, but of course it is fundamentally essential that a bronchoscope of suitable outside diameter is chosen for each patient (Table 3-1).

We have not yet found a use for the flexible laryngopharyngoscope or for the flexible bronchoscopes currently available.

There are a variety of small-diameter Hopkins fiberoptic telescopes whose light may be directed straight ahead or at various angles. The finest of these telescopes are 2.8 mm and the next range are 4.0 mm in external diameter. The telescopes are used constantly in the larynx, tracheobronchial tree, and esophagus and allow an excellent view. They are advantageous for careful evaluation of the laryngeal ventricles, the vocal cords, and the subglottic larynx. Telescopes with a viewing angle of 0°, 30°, and 70° can be conveniently used to examine not only all parts of the larynx with previously unavailable clarity and precision but also the tracheobronchial tree.

The advent of endolaryngeal microsurgery utilizing a self-retaining laryngoscope and the microlaryngeal instruments used in conjunction with the Zeiss operating microscope has revolutionized the ability to perform precise laryngeal manipulations. The laryngoscope is supported by a special holding rod, the foot of which rests on a table over the patient (never on the patient's chest where it might restrict respiratory movements; see Figure 3-3). The surgeon adjusts the microscope and proceeds to work with both hands.

Clinical application of the carbon dioxide laser in the field of surgery of the aerodigestive tract enables the surgeon to direct a laser beam accurately into any part of the field seen with the microscope (Figure 3-3). We have used the microsurgical laser in pediatric laryngology for several years and have found that the advantages of the instrument make it suitable for precise vaporization of laryngeal papillomata with constant visual control of the beam, virtual absence of bleeding, less reactive edema, and little postoperative pain. It is not uncommon, however, to require use of small cupped forceps, angled left, right, or upward to remove residual papillomata from difficult areas after laser surgery and in conjunction with it. Besides papillomata we have used the laser for treating congenital webs, acquired stenoses, hemangiomata, lymphangiomata, and selected tumors.

Table 3-1
Guide to Bronchoscope Size

Size Marked on Bronchoscope (mm)	True External Diameter (mm)	Age Range
2.5	4.0	Premature to neonate
3.0	5.0	Neonate to 6 months
3.5	5.7	6 to 18 months
4.0	7.0	18 to 36 months
5.0	7.8	3 to 8 years
6.0	8.2	Over 8 years

If the bronchoscope is tight after it passes the glottic opening the next smaller bronchoscope should be used to minimize subglottic trauma.

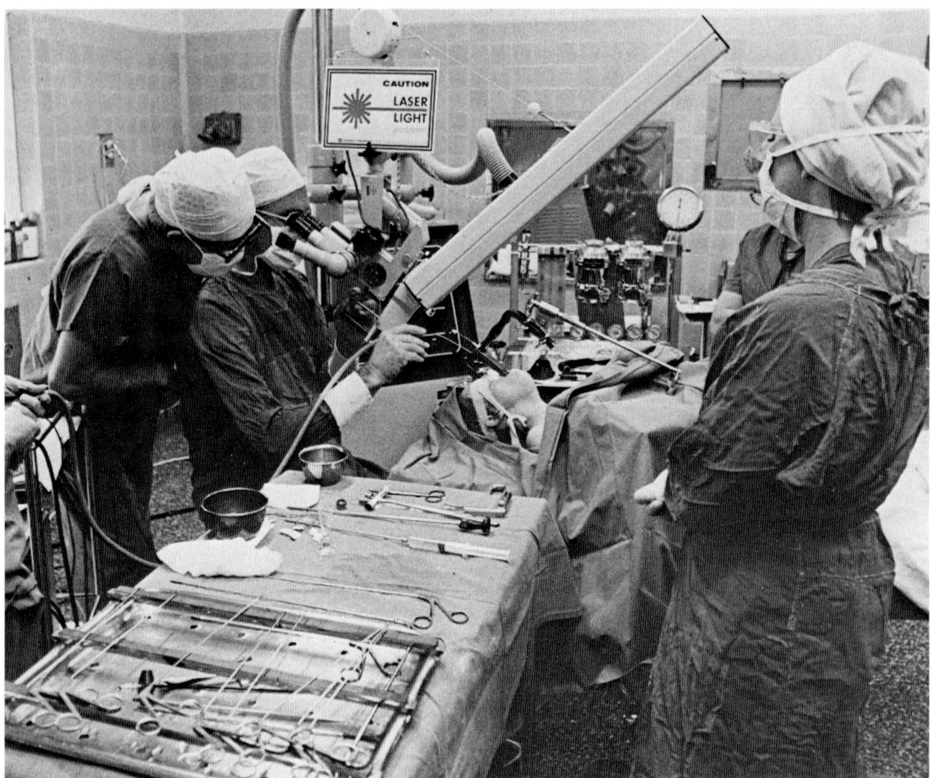

Figure 3-3. *The operating room system for use of the microsurgical laryngeal laser. The self-retaining microlaryngoscope rests on a support over the patient's chest, and the surgeon has both hands free for operative manipulation.*

Method of Laryngoscopy

The infant larynx (see Figure 2, p. v) differs in appearance and structure from the larynx of the adult. The infant larynx is higher: at birth it is located at the level of C4; it descends to C5 by about 6 years of age, and to C6 or C7 by the early teens. The infant larynx is smaller in size and smaller in proportion to the rest of the body than the adult. There is a more acute angle between the glottis and the epiglottis, and the larynx tilts downward and anteriorly, allowing the epiglottis to fall more readily over the laryngeal inlet. The larynx may be said to be under the base of the tongue. Because the infant larynx is higher, softer, and more easily displaced during manipulation it is more easily irritated and there is a greater tendency to spasm. The softer, more flabby and less rigid supporting tissues, especially the less rigid cartilagenous framework, predisposes to collapse of the larynx during the changing pressure of the respiratory cycle. Enlargement of the laryngopharyngeal space during inspiration and constriction during expiration is more conspicuous during respiratory obstruction, and then the pharyngeal upper respiratory chamber is often seen to be expanded and dilated. It must be emphasized that most acute obstructions in infants and children occur in the vital subglottic area. The diameter of the infant larynx is smaller in the subglottic region than at the glottic opening, and serious edema is more easily induced in the infant larynx because of the loosely attached epithelium and underlying connective tissue. Irritation and edema due to inflammation or trauma cause rapid swelling in the subglottic space, which is bounded by the rigid ring of the cricoid cartilage.

These basic considerations underlie some of the difficulties of direct laryngoscopy in infants and children.

Direct Laryngoscopy

Except in emergencies direct laryngoscopy is performed in an operating room with full facilities available. These should include an alternate light source, a full range of bronchoscopes, suckers, and ancillary instruments together with facilities for providing an artificial airway. The latter include not only the range of bronchoscopes but a suitable range of endotracheal tubes (with appropriate introducers) and facilities for emergency or elective tracheotomy.

Endoscopic examination of the larynx, pharynx, and tracheobronchial tree can be successfully and safely performed at any age, if necessary, even in premature infants weighing 1 kg or less. The hospital must have the necessary equipment for investigation, together with experienced anesthetic and endoscopic personnel. A fully staffed postoperative recovery ward and intensive care area with facilities to immediately recognize, diagnose, and manage potential complications is essential. A multidisciplinary approach with close cooperation between the pediatric physician, endoscopist, anesthesiologist, and others involved in the child's care is essential.

All instruments to be introduced into the airway must be sterilized, but the procedure itself is regarded as "clean" rather than surgically aseptically sterile. Naturally, sucker tips or forceps passed into the larynx or tracheobronchial tree are kept uncontaminated. Gentleness and an appreciation of the delicate structures being handled must always be foremost in the mind of the endoscopist.

The infant or child lies flat on his back on a regular, horizontal operating table. There is no necessity for a special head rest or for any form of head restraint. No assistant is needed to hold or move the head (Figure 3-4).

As outlined above, general anesthesia supplemented by local anesthesia is used for endoscopic examination of the respiratory tract in infants and children. The surgeon and anesthesiologist must have a full understanding of what each is doing and of the potential complications in the particular patient being examined. The spontaneous respiration technique or anesthesia allows the opportunity for careful and unhurried observation of the dynamics of the laryngeal apparatus, especially of vocal cord movement.

The first phase of the examination is begun when the anesthesia reaches the required depth using the face mask. Local anesthetic has already been applied and the child continues to breathe spontaneously while the laryngoscope is introduced. Care is taken to retract the upper and lower lips to protect them from trauma and to avoid injury to the teeth. The laryngoscope is passed along the side of the tongue, at first in front of the epiglottis and later behind it to adequately expose the endolarynx by lifting the laryngoscope with the left hand (Figure 3-5). A lever action is never used. The head and neck are flexed as the laryngoscope is first inserted and then extended more as the glottis is exposed.

Although direct laryngoscopy is principally to examine the larynx, other anatomic

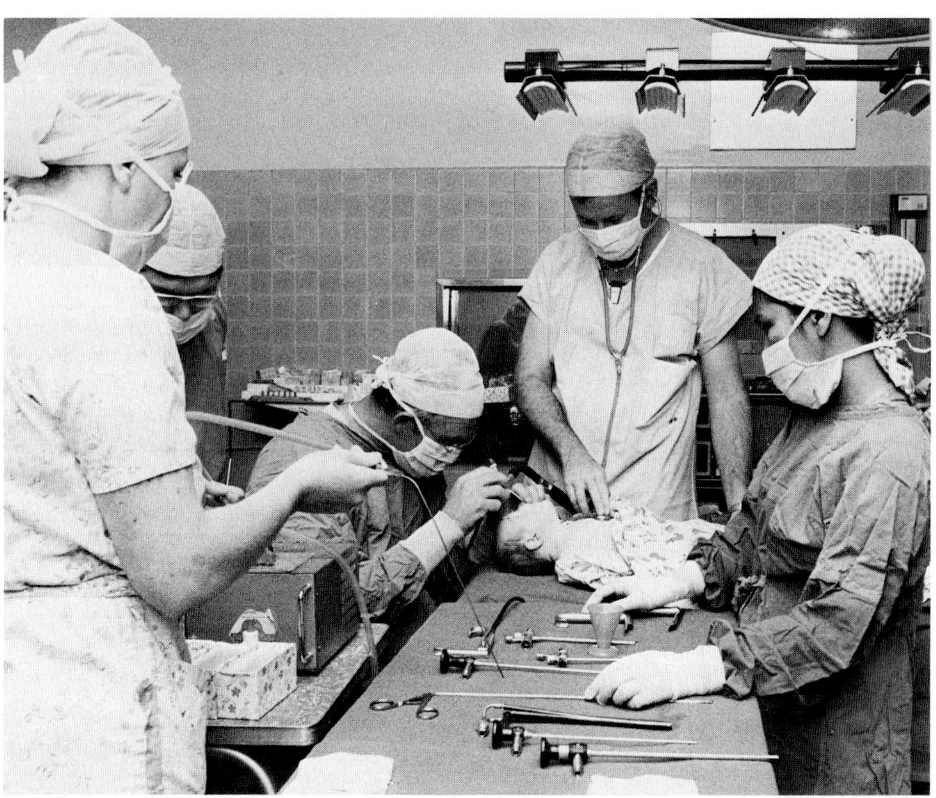

Figure 3-4. *The technique for diagnostic endoscopy. A range of endoscopes suitable for the child's size and age have been selected; suction is readily available for use; the anesthesiologist monitors the patient's respiration and heartbeat. The operating room personnel work together as a team.*

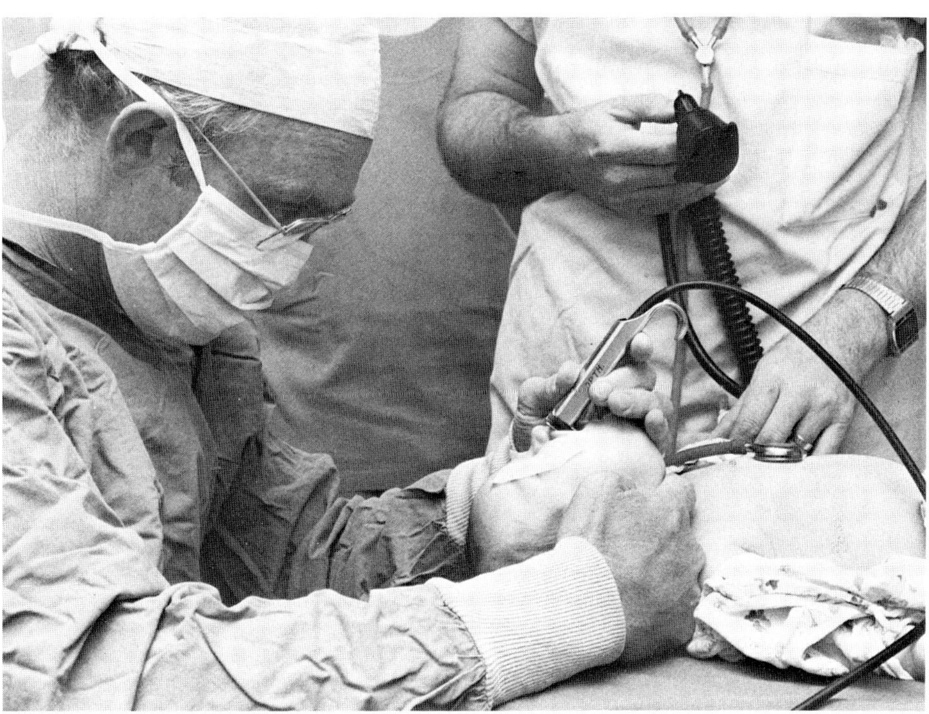

Figure 3-5. *Direct laryngoscopy with the child breathing spontaneously. Note the index finger on the child's neck to manipulate the laryngeal structures for ready visualization.*

areas should always be evaluated; these include the oropharynx, the base of the tongue and the valleculae, the piriform fossae, the postcricoid region, the epiglottis, the arytenoids, the false cords, the ventricles, the vocal cords including the anterior and posterior commissure, and the subglottic region and upper trachea. External pressure and manipulation of the larynx using finger or fingers on the neck (Figure 3-5) with gentle counterpressure from the distal beak of the laryngoscope will rotate or displace the larynx sufficiently to make one or other side of the endolarynx or subglottic region more prominent and easier to visualize.

Initially, then, these areas are examined macroscopically with the naked eye, with the laryngoscope in the left hand and a fine suction tube in the right.

Anesthesia is then continued and deepened with the face mask until the second phase of the procedure using various telescopes can be performed and preparatory to introducing the bronchoscope later.

Laryngoscopy with Telescopes

The laryngoscope is again introduced, and now more detailed evaluation is made using the Hopkins rigid telescopes, straight-ahead and angled. The straight-ahead telescope is used in every case to evaluate the anatomic structures, to inspect the mucosa, and to give a clear magnified image of any pathologic condition present (Figure 3-6). The angled telescopes, 30° and 70°, are especially useful for examination in the laryngeal ventricles, for the anterior and posterior commissure, and for the subglottic region. In most cases this is a more convenient means of performing

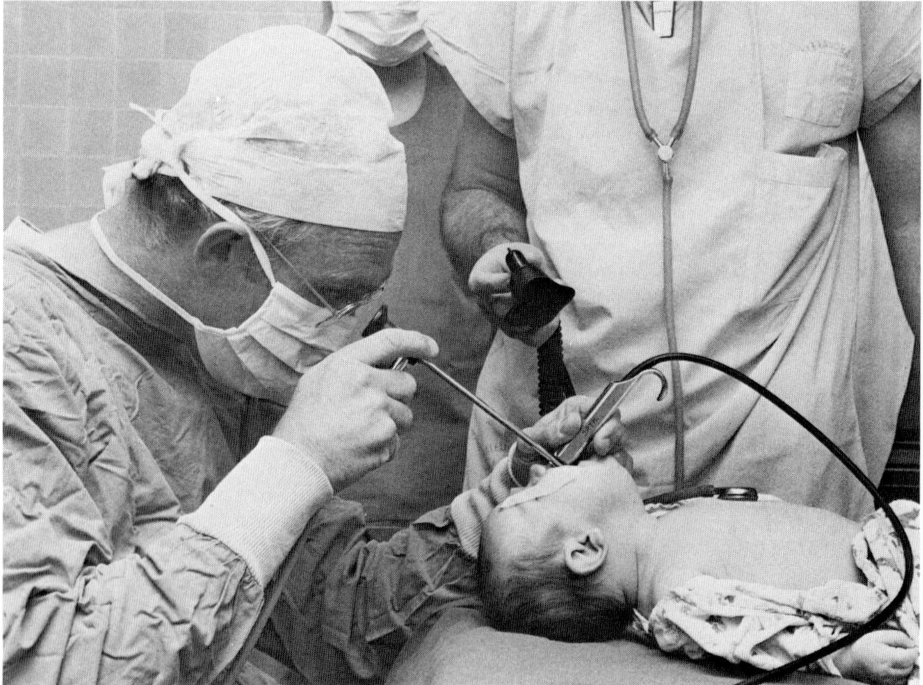

Figure 3-6. *Laryngoscopy with the Hopkins telescope. Closer examination of the structures can be made with bright illumination, a clear image, and minimal trauma.*

a thorough examination than using the specially constructed operating laryngoscopes for microsurgery that, once fixed by the laryngoscope holder, somewhat limit manipulation and complete visualization of the laryngeal structures other than the glottic opening itself. Nevertheless the microlaryngeal technique is essential when the findings indicate that surgery is necessary. We regularly proceed from direct laryngoscopy with telescopes to microlaryngoscopy for endolaryngeal microsurgery.

In other words, the two methods are combined so that a preliminary survey of the oropharynx and laryngopharynx is accomplished with the hand-held laryngoscope and Hopkins telescope and then a suitably sized endolaryngeal microsurgical speculum is placed and held in position by a self-retaining jack, ready for the appropriate surgical procedure.

Microlaryngoscopy

Microlaryngeal surgery is now firmly established as part of modern laryngology. A 400-mm objective lens is used and the beam splitter allows adaptation of the Zeiss microscope for an observer eyepiece. Microsurgery offers the advantages of variable magnification, brilliant illumination, binocular vision, and use of a self-retaining and self-supporting laryngoscope. In this way microlaryngoscopy allows thorough examination for accurate diagnosis and for precise surgical treatment, more recently with the carbon dioxide laser. Nevertheless, there are some disadvantages.

A general anesthetic technique requiring a standard endotracheal tube does not allow adequate exposure for the surgical procedure, as the presence of the endotracheal tube obstructs the surgeon's view. Anesthetic methods without a tube or with a modified tube are preferable for the surgeon but in some cases are not so acceptable to the anesthesiologist, as there may not be sufficient control of ventilation. There are many techniques of anesthesia for examination or manipulation within the larynx, some developed since the advent of microsurgery of the larynx. The techniques generally come into one or more of the following groups:

1. No endotracheal tube. Spontaneous respiration with insufflation of oxygen, nitrous oxide, and halothane either through a nasopharyngeal tube (Figure 3-7) or through a small tube incorporated in the laryngoscope (Figure 3-8) is the commonest technique to maintain stable anesthesia. Another uses a venturi jet proximally in the lumen of the laryngoscope but has the disadvantage of drying the larynx, blowing blood or papilloma into the trachea, and of causing movement of the larynx that might distract or interrupt the surgeon.
2. A modified endotracheal tube. A small-diameter standard endotracheal tube (Figure 3-9) is used with high-flow oxygen insufflation, or some other modification of an endotracheal tube with the patient paralyzed or the patient breathing spontaneously. Some techniques utilize a catheter with the venturi jet technique. We favor the use of the "Benjamin jet tube"[1] (Figure 3-10) for microlaryngeal surgery in patients over the age of 5 years when a relaxant technique is required. A venturi jet system is attached to the proximal end of the recently developed Benjet tube. The distal end of the tube is positioned in the midtrachea and the four soft plastic flanges maintain it in its central position, thus preventing trauma to the tracheal wall and ensuring even distribution

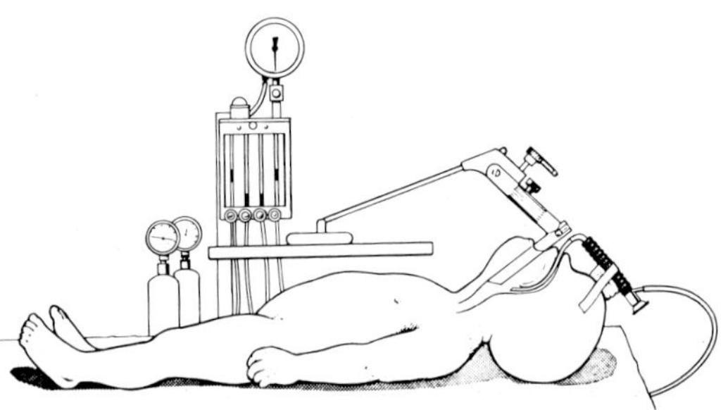

Figure 3-7. *Nasopharyngeal insufflation of oxygen, nitrous oxide, and halothane with spontaneous respiration.*

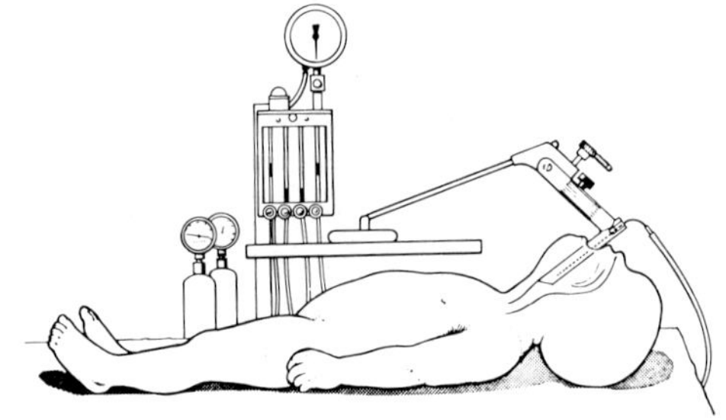

Figure 3-8. *Insufflation directly into the lumen of the laryngoscope through a long, wide-bore French's blood airway needle, again using spontaneous respiration with oxygen, nitrous oxide, and halothane.*

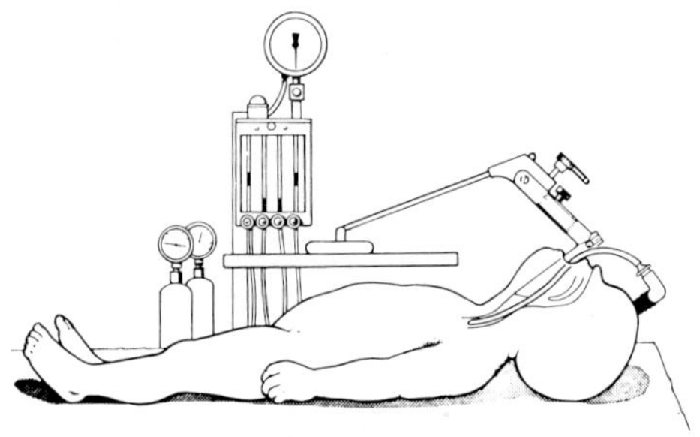

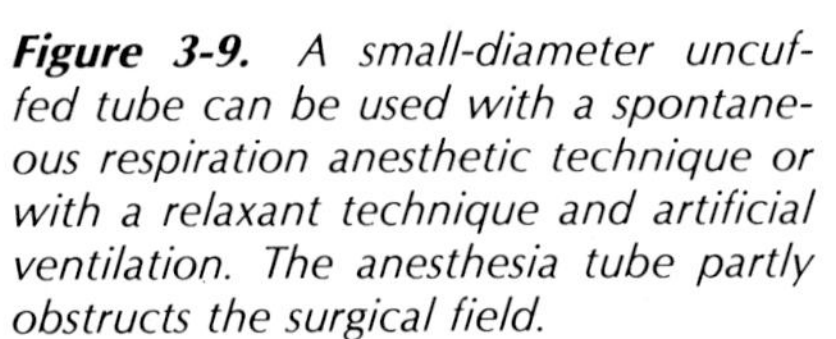

Figure 3-9. *A small-diameter uncuffed tube can be used with a spontaneous respiration anesthetic technique or with a relaxant technique and artificial ventilation. The anesthesia tube partly obstructs the surgical field.*

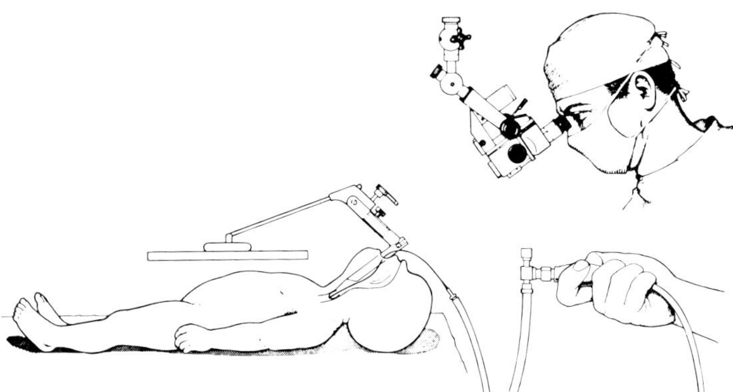

Figure 3-10. *The "Benjamin jet tube" (2.8 mm O.D.) used with the venturi jet technique in a paralyzed patient. Suitable for children over 5 years of age.*

of the gases. The outside diameter of the tube for pediatric use is 2.8 mm and it lies conveniently and unobtrusively in the posterior commissure of the larynx, allowing the surgeon an excellent view of the surgical field. If necessary it can be displaced into the anterior commissure so that the surgeon can work in the posterior part of the glottic opening.

3. Anesthesia may be delivered via a tracheotomy (Figure 3-11). This applies only in patients where tracheotomy is required because of the nature of the congenital or acquired lesion itself. The tracheotomy facilitates anesthesia and gives ideal operating conditions for the surgeon.

The anesthetic requirements for laryngeal microsurgery include simplicity, rapid induction yet prompt recovery, an immobile and unobstructed operative field, no restriction on time, control of secretions, prevention of aspiration, and safe use of the laser. These ideals must, however, be compatible with maximal safety and minimal patient discomfort.

There are many patterns of laryngoscopes available for microsurgery, but the principle embodied in each system is the same: there should be a wide proximal end to allow binocular vision and adequate entry of both the suction and the instruments so that two hands are available for endolaryngeal surgery. The distal end is

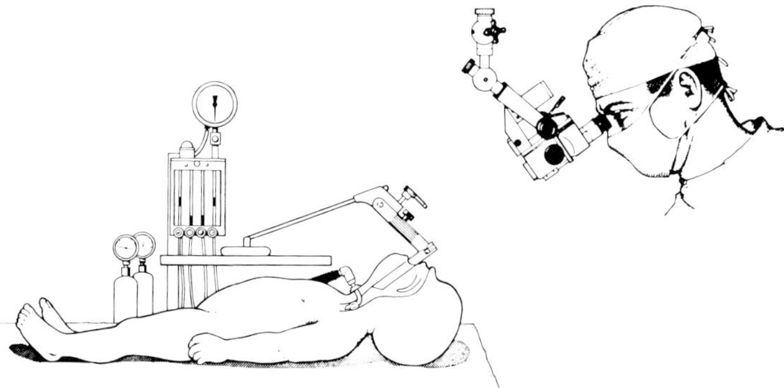

Figure 3-11. *Anesthesia via a tracheotomy tube allows ideal conditions both for the surgical procedure in the larynx and for control of anesthesia by the anesthesiologist.*

of a suitable size to expose the infant larynx yet not be traumatic. Some form of illumination in the laryngoscope is necessary for its introduction, but this can be discarded once the operating microscope is in place and providing illumination. The self-retaining supporting rod should rest on an over-table rather than on the patient's chest, where it might restrict respiration.

Microsurgical instruments include a range of suction tubes, cupped forceps, scissors, grasping forceps, suction-cautery probe, and various knives and hooks.

Laser Surgery

The most exciting and useful advance in recent years is application of the carbon dioxide laser in this field (see Figure 3-3). Tissue can be removed precisely with minimal bleeding and lessened postoperative reaction. An aiming beam indicates the exact treatment site, and with a micromanipulator that is mounted on the microscope each laser exposure can be precisely placed. The instrument is particularly suitable for vaporization of laryngeal papillomata with constant visual control of the beam; there is little or no bleeding, so that treatment of papillomata on multiple sites can usually be performed at one operation. Without the laser (using forceps and other instruments), bleeding tends to obscure the operative site and fewer papillomata can be safely removed. When the tumors are not removed at one operation they are removed at the next or the next or the next. There should be no hesitation to perform multiple operations for this condition.

Certain special precautions must be taken when the laser is in use. Combustible anesthetic gases must be avoided, care should be exercised not to ignite the anesthetic tube if one is being used, the beam should not be allowed to bounce off shiny metal surfaces, and the eyes of the patient and all others in the operating theatre must be protected. At times the beam can be bounced off tiny metal mirrors made specially for the purpose should there be lesions in difficult anatomical sites such as the laryngeal ventricle or the subglottic region. The laser energy is absorbed by moisture, and use of a small, moist cottonoid will protect adjacent tissues.

Laryngoscopic Findings

The diameter of the subglottic region should be assessed in every case, not only in patients being assessed for suspected congenital subglottic stenosis. With knowledge of the outside diameter of the bronchoscope (Table 3-1) that comfortably passes through the subglottic region, the internal diameter of the cricoid can be calibrated and recorded for future reference.

A confident diagnosis of laryngomalacia can be made only by direct examination. Not only will complete endoscopic examination positively confirm the diagnosis but the possibility of any associated abnormality in the tracheobronchial tree will be excluded. The characteristic changes of laryngomalacia are seen during the initial laryngoscopy or later as the administration of anesthesia is discontinued. The distal tip of the laryngoscope blade is placed in the vallecula at the base of the tongue above and in front of the epiglottis as the patient is regaining muscular tone and movement. The epiglottis in laryngomalacia is typically abnormal, being tall, narrow, and folded upon itself so that its lateral margins lie close together. The omega-shaped epiglottis appears to be curled and tubular. The aryepiglottic folds and arytenoids are tall, thin, and flaccid, appearing lax and redundant, and are sucked into the larynx on each inspiration. On expiration they are blown upward and outward so that expiration is totally unimpeded. When the epiglottis and aryepiglottic folds are splinted out with the laryngoscope above the vocal cords, the airway obstruction and stridor is immediately corrected.

Congenital infantile subglottic hemangioma has an appearance that is sufficiently characteristic for an experienced observer to make a macroscopic diagnosis without biopsy, especially if there are associated cutaneous hemangiomata. The lesion is usually localized to the subglottic region on one side as a sessile, fairly firm, compressible pink or bluish lesion poorly delineated from the surrounding tissues. Biopsy may be performed where the diagnosis is uncertain, taking due precaution to maintain the airway in the unlikely event that there is excessive bleeding.

Care must be exercised with the initial anesthesia and examination in patients with laryngeal papillomatosis. Although airway obstruction may not be apparent or may appear to be minimal at preoperative assessment and before anesthesia is commenced, it is common for obstruction to occur as the depth of anesthesia is increased. In these patients it may be wise to commence examination in the operating room with the laryngoscope and the bronchoscope readily available. Laryngoscopy at the first examination should be for biopsy removal of a large bulk of the growths on one side of the larynx (see Figure 3, p. v). This gives histopathologic confirmation of the diagnosis and establishes a satisfactory glottic opening for subsequent operations in diffuse cases. Care must be taken at all times during surgery to prevent adhesions and subsequent web formation at the anterior commissure. The growths have a predilection for involvement of the anterior commissure at the vocal cord level, and patients who have had multiple operations are likely to develop an anterior glottic web.

A small congenital glottic web may present as a weak or hoarse cry, and a larger web with partial airway obstruction or atypically prolonged and repeated croup. The web is at the anterior part of the larynx, and it is important to assess not only its anteroposterior dimensions but also its thickness (see Figure 5, p. v). This is usually seen on the preoperative xeroradiogram, but further information is gained by examination of the glottic and subglottic region with angled telescopes. There is often a congenital subglottic stenosis in association with larger webs. A very rare web is that producing congenital interarytenoid fixation. There is a posterior web in the interarytenoid region so that an erroneous diagnosis of bilateral vocal cord paralysis may be made because the vocal cords are seen to be in adduction. Abduction is prevented by the posterior interarytenoid web's causing fixation, with a tight band of tissue fixing the arytenoids to one another.

The Pierre Robin syndrome of micrognathia, retroposed tongue, and cleft palate is associated with a varying degree of upper airway obstruction. Laryngoscopy is necessary only where the possibility of other congenital airway abnormalities must be excluded or where endotracheal intubation is undertaken to provide a temporary artificial airway. In these cases it is difficult to visualize the larynx, and cooperation between the anesthesiologist and the endoscopist is especially valuable. A complete range of endoscopes is necessary, including, of course, the Holinger anterior commissure laryngoscope.

An inhaled foreign body is usually found in the tracheobronchial tree, but some foreign bodies lodge in the larynx, usually in the subglottic region, sometimes in the supraglottic larynx or between the vocal cords themselves. A piece of eggshell inhaled by an infant will impinge in the sagittal plane and can be detected radiologically by an anteroposterior film. A husky, weak, or absent cry, atypical croup, and persistent wheezing and airway obstruction should all suggest the possibility of a laryngeal foreign body; and if the presence of a difficult foreign body in this area is recognized before endoscopy, in some cases it is safer to perform tracheotomy using face mask inhalational anesthesia or local anesthesia. Anesthesia can then be continued via the tracheotomy during removal of the foreign body. A certain amount of ingenuity may be required with this problem of removing awkward objects. A foreign body in the laryngeal area should always be treated with great respect, as the technique of removal is critical.

A cyst in the larynx or pharynx large enough to cause airway obstruction is not common; but where there is a laryngeal or pharyngeal cyst, partial airway obstruction may suddenly become total during induction of anesthesia or commencement of instrumentation and a critical situation may occur. The lateral airways x-ray or xeroradiogram should have revealed the presence of such a problem before it occurs, and the surgeon should be alerted and fully prepared, for example, to decompress the cyst by sucking out its contents or by incising it.

The endoscopist must be careful in assessing vocal cord movement. It is easy to mistake a vocal cord paralysis if pressure from the laryngoscope blade by the direction in which it is introduced suggests a false diagnosis of right vocal cord paralysis.

It is now generally accepted that neonates withstand prolonged endotracheal intubation with relatively little morbidity or serious damage to the larynx. This is especially so in a neonatal intensive care ward with optimal nursing and correct choice of a tube of sufficiently small diameter that it can move freely in the subglottic region with a suitable air leak around the tube. Endoscopy is performed in these patients only if, after extubation, there are indications of a complication such as subglottic edema, persisting airway obstruction, or a weak or husky cry (see Figure 6, p. v).

In older children up to the age of 8 or 10 years where there is no serious laryngeal pathologic condition causing airway obstruction we maintain "prolonged" intubation with a tube that has no cuff for up to a week before the situation is reviewed. Then, if necessary, endoscopic examination is performed and a decision made as to whether tracheotomy should be performed or intubation should continue. Serious endoscopic findings suggesting the need to discontinue intubation include circumferential ulceration in the subglottic region; ulceration down to the cartilage, especially through the perichondrium covering the lamina of the cricoid cartilage; proliferative granulation tissue, and signs of soft tissue infection.

Thus, endoscopic evaluation at the appropriate time can assist in the decision as to whether a patient requiring ventilatory support should continue to have an endotracheal tube as the artificial airway or whether tracheotomy should be considered as an alternative.

Occasionally the larynx may be difficult or even impossible to visualize or the anterior commissure may not be seen clearly with the regular laryngoscope. The specially designed Holinger anterior commissure infant laryngoscope will invariably be superior and even in extremely distorted and congenitally abnormal larynges this instrument will enable the examination to be completed successfully. The larynx may be difficult to expose in Pierre Robin syndrome; in Treacher-Collins syndrome; in Crouzon's disease; in babies with marked micrognathia, where there has been distortion of the neck and pharynx from external trauma or burn contracture; in ankylosis of the cervical spine; in limitation of movement of the temporomandibular joint; or in other rare congenital anomalies such as congenital interarytenoid fixation.

Laryngeal Photography

Photographic documentation of laryngeal, tracheal, or bronchial disease is now possible on a routine basis using the Storz equipment. The rigid Hopkins telescopes give clear color illumination so that 35-mm single frame still photography, cinephotography, or closed-circuit television with video cassette recording can be made with great reliability and reproducibility.

We have used the miniature Storz lightweight motorized endocamera for many years to obtain color transparency photographs of the respiratory tract including the nasopharynx, pharynx, larynx, trachea, bronchi, and esophagus. We use the Storz electronic flash generator in combination with the various rigid Hopkins telescopes. We use 200 ASA Kodak Ektachrome film for routine procedures but 400 ASA Kodak Ektachrome for photography of the nasopharynx through the 120° retrograde telescope.

Some form of antifog solution is needed to prevent misting of the telescope; we use Ultrastop. Initially some practice is required to be sure that the field of view is exactly central in the telescope and in the sagittal plane. This is important for orientation by the viewer and to compare the right with the left side. Some experience is also required in judging whether to use setting 1, 2, or 3 on the electronic flash generator. These settings vary the exposure time of the flash and must be changed according to the distance between the distal end of the telescope and the area to be photographed.

Cinephotography requires the use of the xenon light source for extrabright illumination and the Wittmoser multiarticulated arm. We use a 16-mm movie camera with automatic exposure control. One point of technique is that the proximal arm of the Wittmoser must be rotated by the movie operator to maintain the field of view in the anteroposterior diameter.

Precautions and Complications

In those cases where there is airway obstruction, anesthesia and endoscopic instrumentation may precipitate total obstruction and should therefore be attempted only if the diagnosis cannot be made in any other way or if endoscopic surgical treatment of the obstruction is necessary. If such a problem is anticipated anesthesia is started in the operating room with the endoscopic instruments functional and with instruments for a tracheotomy readily at hand.

Twin flexible fiberoptic light cables allow the laryngoscope and the bronchoscope to be used simultaneously, adding a safety margin where a bronchoscope is needed to provide an airway at short notice. Reliable suction must be available at all times.

Special precautions during laser surgery have already been outlined.

Many other safety factors should be considered. These include respiratory depression by injudicious administration of drugs; maintenance of a small baby's body temperature by minimizing heat loss; careful selection of instruments to cause minimal tissue trauma; gentle handling of tissues especially in the vulnerable subglottic area; minimization of mucosal trauma with as little disruption as possible of the respiratory tract mucociliary mechanism; optimal humidification of the inspired air; adequate systemic hydration, using intravenous fluids whenever necessary; as little handling of neonates as possible; aspiration of secretions and blood during and at the completion of examination; adequate facilities in a fully equipped recovery ward for the recognition and treatment of potential complications; and the ready availability of expert medical resuscitation at all times.

Most patients have recovered muscular tone and are awake from the anesthetic within a short time of having been returned to the recovery room. After the use of topical local anesthesia we do not allow oral fluids for a minimum of 3 hours.

The effects of anesthesia and of the endoscopic examination are necessarily traumatic, even in a minor degree, because of the instruments that are introduced, the trauma to the surface mucosa of the respiratory tract, the drying effect of the anesthetic gases and of atropine, and, in infants, the loss of body heat.

Edema in the subglottic region of the larynx may be caused by excessive manipulation, passage of too large a bronchoscope, or repeated or prolonged manipulations. Subglottic edema is manifested as a croupy cough, stridor, and increasing airway obstruction that may progress over some hours in severe cases. Naturally, careful technique will reduce the incidence to a minimum; but should this complication occur, adequate hydration of the patient, humidification of the inspired air, and in selected cases administration of high doses of steroids are the methods of treatment. Humidification of the inspired air is most beneficial in maintaining a warm, moist respiratory mucosa. The mucociliary mechanism can be affected by drying of the mucosa or trauma from instrumentation and suction, leading to diminished efficiency of coughing.

Rough handling of the instruments may lead to loosening or dislodgement of teeth, laceration of the lips or gums, and bleeding from mucosal tears.

References

1. Benjamin B, Gronow D: A new tube for microlaryngeal surgery. Anaesth Intensive Care 7:258, 1979

Bronchoscopy

CHAPTER 4

Stephen L. Gans

Bronchoesophagology is the study of two lines of communication on which human life depends for its supplies—the air tubes and the food passages. A most important part of this study is the direct examination of these organs for diagnosis and for certain aspects of treatment. It is the intent of this chapter (Bronchoscopy) and the next (Esophagoscopy) to bring this part of the subject into view, particularly in light of the new instruments and techniques that have refined the art.

For years most bronchoscopy has been done with an open tube with a light at one end or the other. It has been possible for a few particularly gifted and skilled bronchologists to obtain a direct view of the anatomy and pathology of the tracheobronchial tree. Even in their hands, however, examination was often inadequate, prolonged, repeated, and even abandoned. Because of this, the procedure was frequently hazardous, errors were made, and teaching and learning of the art were difficult.

The development of miniature telescopes combined with fiberoptic lighting (see Chapter 1) has increased the safety, accuracy, and indications for this procedure. The superior view provides both a sharp, magnified, and wide-angle image, making orientation easy and quick, and sufficient light for photodocumentation, television, and split-image teaching attachments. At the same time there is enough space remaining in the bronchoscope sheath for adequate ventilation and/or anesthesia and for the use of a number of manipulating instruments. For all of these reasons it is now possible for a surgeon with reasonable dexterity, and surgical and anatomical experience with the involved organs, to become proficient in this important field.

Some individuals have used the *flexible* bronchoscopes, but the small size of the trachea and the lack of ventilating sufficiency has limited the use of these instruments in the pediatric age group. Furthermore, the view suffers by comparison, and the capabilities for instrumental manipulation are minimal.

Indications and Clinical Features

As stated by Benjamin in Chapter 3, bronchoscopy is an extension and integral part of laryngoscopy, and many of the clinical conditions and symptoms indicating each procedure are the same or similar. The reader is referred to Chapter 3 as an introduction to this subject.

It should be emphasized that *acute inflammatory disease* seldom requires endoscopic investigation although it may cause serious obstruction. Differential diagnosis of this condition from that of a foreign body impacted in the trachea or upper esophagus can usually be made by the history of a more acute onset and of possible ingestion of some object, and special x-rays or xeroradiograms may be very helpful.

Tracheal narrowing due to compression, collapse, or stenosis is usually associated with an inspiratory stridor, sometimes with an expiratory component, and often with a barking cough. *Compression* of the tracheobronchial tree may be due to mediastinal tumors, bronchogenic cysts, esophageal duplication cysts, crushing injury, or vascular rings (see Figure 10, p. v). In addition to endoscopy, other studies are helpful and indicated.

Tracheomalacia is best evaluated by endoscopy and, of course, differentiated from other lesions collapsing the trachea. Growth of the child and the size of the trachea most often compensates for this defect in time. Superimposed inflammation is a problem that complicates the partial obstruction. In the most severe instances, tracheostomy may be indicated.

There are several varieties and degrees of *stenosis* demanding endoscopic evaluation and, frequently, treatment. A thin congenital web or band can be easily dilated or incised. Longer segments of congenital tracheal stenosis may require dilatation or resection. Postinflammatory, postintubation, and posttracheostomy obstructions present a large gamut of problems sometimes taxing the patience, skill, and ingenuity of the surgeon as well as the response, reaction, and even survival of the patient. Most important is the intial endoscopic evaluation of the severity and extent of the problem. Then, sometimes, only observation or minor dilatation is the proper approach. More severe granuloma or scar formation may require dilatation, resection (electrosurgery, cryosurgery, laser surgery), or external plastic or resectional therapy.

A *laryngotracheoesophageal* cleft may involve only the larynx with a cleft between the arytenoids or may extend all the way to the thoracic inlet. In order to determine the proper approach for repair, precise evaluation of the anatomic defect is necessary and can only be done by direct laryngobronchoscopic examination.

We have found it quite safe and useful to bronchoscopically examine each infant before repair of *esophageal atresia with tracheoesophageal fistula*, either preceding the definitive operation or before the first procedure in the staged methods. In a few seconds we can localize the tracheal, carinal, or bronchial opening of the fistula (see Figure 9, p. v) and can also eliminate the presence of, or indeed discover, a proximal segment fistula.

The symptoms of choking or coughing with feedings, excessive tracheal secretions, and recurrent atelectasis or pneumonitis should direct attention to the possibility of an *N-type (H-type*) tracheoesophageal fistula*.[1] The difficulties and inconsistencies of previously described methods of making this diagnosis have been laid to rest by the superior capabilities of modern telescopic endoscopes. The fistula is best seen through the trachea. After introduction of the bronchoscope, orientation is quick, and the opening is identified and inspected. Very often the fistula can be cannulated with a Fogarty or ureteral catheter that can be left in place if immediate repair is planned (Figure 4-1). In this way the fistula is accurately located (neck or chest), and the presence of the catheter allows quick localization by palpation, with limited dissection, accurate and rapid correction, and minimal opportunities for damage to surrounding structures.

The same symptoms indicate the possibility of *recurrent tracheoesophageal fistula* in patients who have had a previous repair of this malformation.[2] A posterior "pit" or "fossa" is seen at the site of a previous tracheal closure, and even sutures may be identified. In many instances the open fistula may be readily appreciated, but sometimes the diagnosis is more difficult because of an erratic fistulous tract that does not allow catheterization. In such cases, a drop or so of methylene blue solution accurately applied through a catheter tip placed directly in the pit or fossa may work its way through such a fistula and appear in the esophagus, where it can be seen by esophagoscopy. Indeed, reports of endoscopic closure of such fistulas have been reported using tissue-adhesive solutions applied directly and accurately with a catheter directed into position by the bronchoscope.[3-5]

Congenital *bronchoenteric or bronchobiliary fistulas*, originating from beneath the diaphragm, have been identified by combinations of endoscopy and radiography. The treatment is closure of the tracheobronchial opening and excision of the tract.

The *removal of viscid tracheobronchial secretions* and the management of atelectasis in infants following major surgical procedures or in pulmonary infections or fibrocystic disease usually do *not* require endoscopy. Occasionally bronchoscopy is helpful for selective therapy to specific lung segments or when nonendoscopic methods fail.

The diagnosis and management of *tracheobronchial foreign bodies* is a subject and art of its own. The variety of aspirated objects is endless, ranging from foods—

*Popularly known as H-type fistula, we believe this entity would be more properly termed *N-type* because the fistula almost always runs diagonally caudad from the trachea to the esophagus.

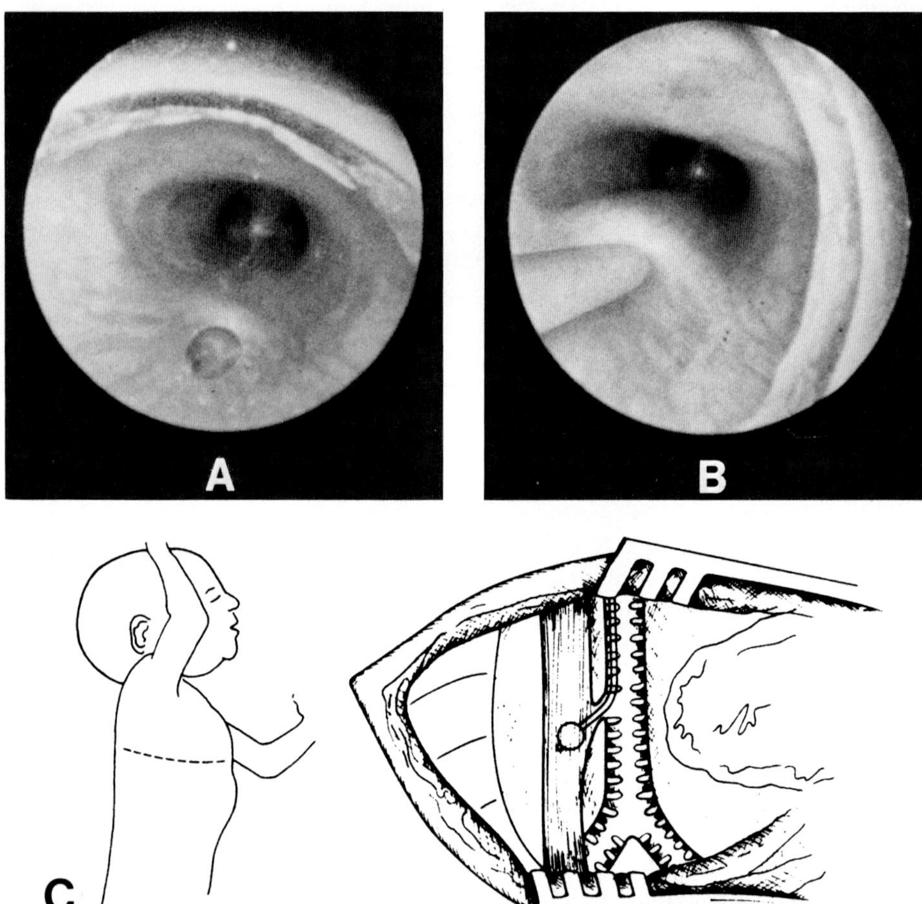

Figure 4-1. *(A) Bronchoscopic demonstration of tracheal opening of N-type tracheoesophageal fistula about 2.5 cm proximal to the carina in a 2300-gm neonate. This is a black-and-white enlargement from a single frame of a color movie. Note the details still retained. (From Gans SL, Johnson RO: Diagnosis and surgical management of "H-type" tracheoesophageal fistula in infants and children. J Pediatr Surg 12:233–236, 1977. With permission.) (B) Fogarty catheter has been passed through the fistula in clear view of the telescope. (C) Thoracic approach, diagrammatically showing the Fogarty catheter with inflated balloon in the esophagus. Minimal dissection is needed to accurately locate and correct the fistula.*

peanuts, carrot or apple pieces, meat, and chicken or fish bones—to crayons, all sorts of hardware, pieces of toys, tin foil, coins, buttons, and teeth. History regarding the nature of the foreign matter may be helpful in establishing the diagnosis.

Symptoms may include spasms of coughing, gagging, choking, and wheezing. As the mucosa and bronchus adjust to this abnormal situation, a symptomless interval may develop, giving a false impression that the object has been coughed out or swallowed. A persistent wheeze or evidence of emphysema or atelectasis calls for further investigation. X-rays document the latter and may demonstrate and localize a radiopaque object. Ultrasound may also be helpful. If there is a serious question or doubt bronchoscopic investigation is indicated. Failure to remove a foreign body may result in pneumonitis, lung abscess, bronchiectasis, pulmonary hemorrhage, or bronchial erosion and perforation.

Equipment

The two optical achievements of recent years, namely the development of the Hopkins rod lens systems and of fiber thread illumination (see Chapter 1), created potentials for pediatric bronchoscopy never before possible. Because of this a complete new set of instruments was designed, developed, and tested[6] that has now become the standard of performance to which all others must be compared.* Bronchoscopic endoscopy in infants and children is now a precise procedure, with instruments sufficiently miniaturized for use in even the smallest patient.

Illumination is provided through fiberoptic cords or cables produced by a variety of cold-light fountains. The light sources range from a small, easily portable unit to more complicated and versatile arrangements featuring everything from multiple outlets, variable power features, and photoflash capabilities to a xenon light source more than adequate for cinephotography and television. (See Figures 2-4 and 2-6.)

An air pump with adjustable pressure is recommended for use with the antifog tubes. This functions very well in most instances to keep the end of the telescope clean and dry. It is also helpful to warm the telescope with warm water (not saline) or to use a drop of sterile surface-tension-reducing solution (Ultrastop).†

The route to the tracheobronchial tree is through the larynx, which indeed in many instances is an integral part of a combined examination. The reader is referred to Chapter 3 for a description of the instruments and equipment recommended for this part of the procedure. In addition, we would like to recommend a special laryngoscope designed by us and made by Storz that greatly facilitates examination of the larynx and introduction of the bronchoscope through the vocal cords. The blade has a spoonlike attachment that prevents the tongue from sliding to one side or the other (Figure 4-2). It also has a built-in channel through which a catheter can extend to the tip for continuous suction, or for intermittent

---

*Karl Storz KG, Tuttlingen, West Germany; Storz Endoscopy–America, Culver City, California.
†Sigmachemie, Vienna.

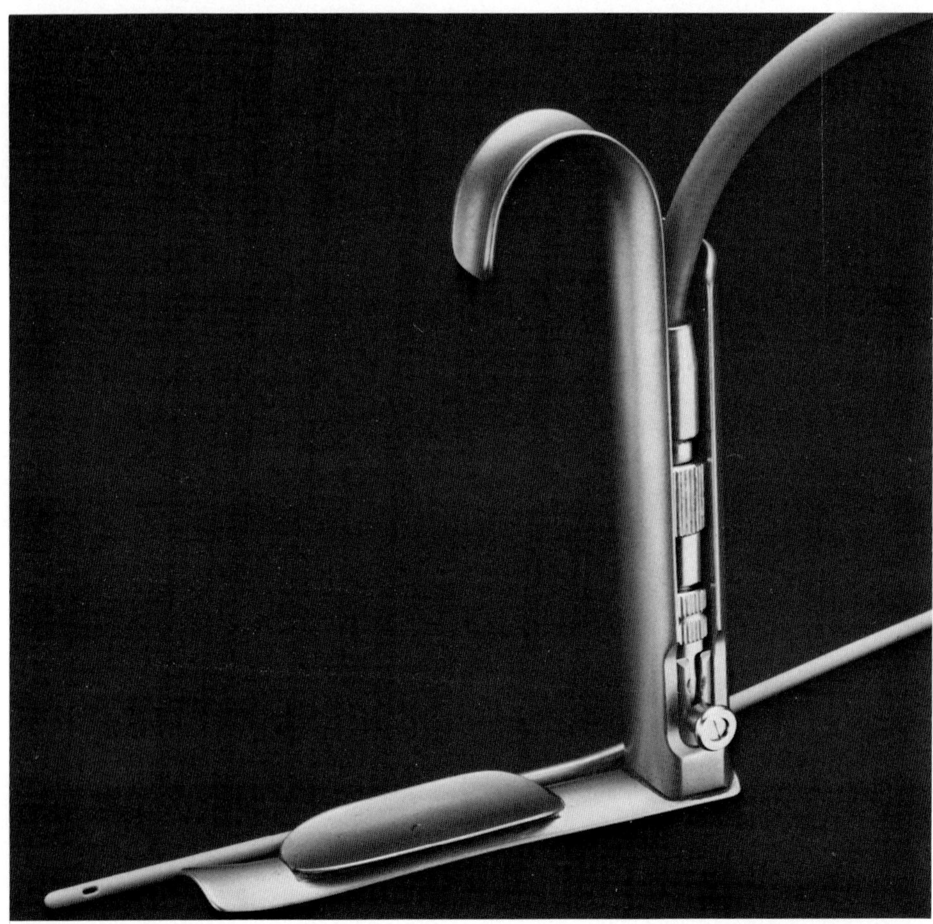

Figure 4-2. *Gans laryngoscope: fiberoptic light cable connected to proximal prism light; spoon-shaped blade; built-in channel through which suction catheter can be moved in or out to an appropriate position.*

suction by a verbal command to an assistant, thus leaving the examiner's other hand free for manipulation and introduction of an airway or bronchoscope.

Figure 4-3 illustrates and provides a list of equipment for use in the neonate or small infant. The dimensions on the bronchoscope sheaths are in millimeters by centimeters. However, the millimeter designation of the diameter traditionally is not accurate either for inside or outside measurement. The exact diameter dimensions are provided in Table 3–1. The 2.5-mm sheath is used without an antifog tube because it barely accommodates the telescope itself; instead, an adaptor or bridge is used to hold the telescope in place. The other sheaths may also be used without antifog tubes as long as the adaptor is interposed.

Figure 4–4 illustrates and lists the instruments for use in intermediate-sized infants and children. Note that there are two different sheath lengths, the 26-cm instrument making an important transition between the mini set and the intermediate set.

Tables 4–1 and 4–2 show the equipment and materials generally needed for bronchoscopy and esophagoscopy.

Table 4-1
General Equipment

Anesthesia or ventilation adaptor
Teaching attachment
Light source (two outlets preferred)
Light cables, two single and one Y-shaped
Air pump with adjustable stream, for antifog
Suction, adjustable as to pressure; intermittent and continuous
Tracheotomy set (available)
X-ray capability (desirable)

Table 4-2
General Supplies

Sterile drapes
Towel clips
Container of warm water (not saline)
Sterile pipestem cleaners, cotton tips, and 4×4 sponges
Curved and straight hemostats
Nasogastric suction catheters

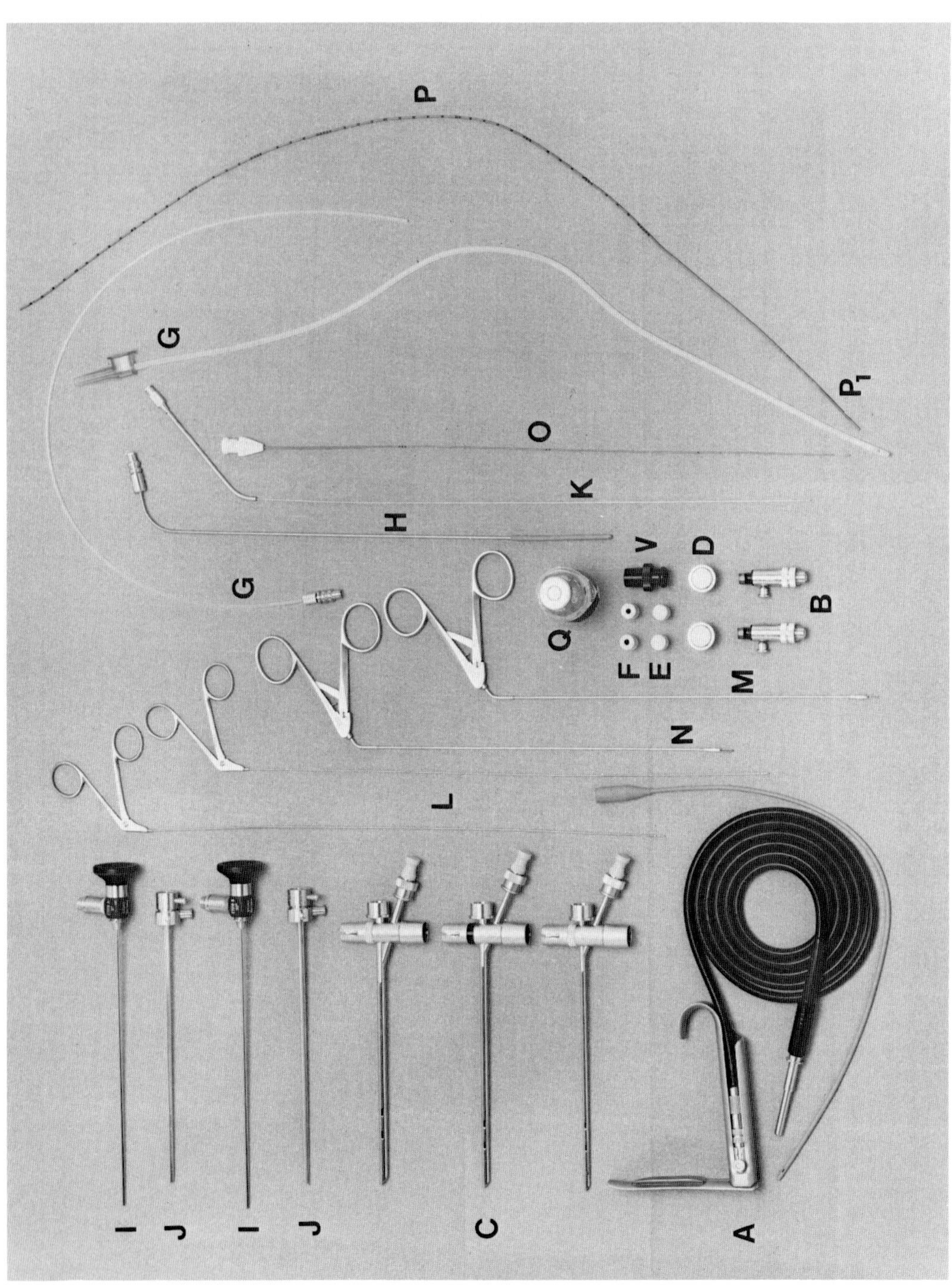

I
J
I
J
C
A
L
N
M
B
D
V
E
F
Q
G
H
K
O
G
P
P_1

Figure 4-3. *Instruments for the neonate or small infant. (A) Laryngoscope with illumination and suction. (B) Prism light deflectors (two). (C) Bronchoscope sheaths: 2.5 mm × 20 cm; 3.0 mm × 20 cm; 4.0 mm × 20 cm. (D) Glass window plugs (two). (E) Nipples without holes (two). (F) Nipples with holes (two). (G) Suction catheters, plastic (two), one to fit instrument channel and a larger one to pass through the sheath. (H) Straight metal suction tubes (two), one with curved rubber tip and one with velvet tip. (I) Storz (Hopkins lens) telescopes: 0° and 30° (70° not illustrated). (J) Antifog tubes for each telescope, and telescopic bridge adaptor (not illustrated) for use when antifog tube is not used. (K) Long injection needle. (L) Biopsy forceps. (M) Alligator forceps. (N) Peanut forceps. (O) Fogarty catheter. (P) Ureteral catheter. (P_1) Wire electrocoagulation tip (not illustrated; see Figure 5-3) to be passed through ureteral catheter. (Q) Ultrastop. (V) Anesthesia or ventilator adaptor.*

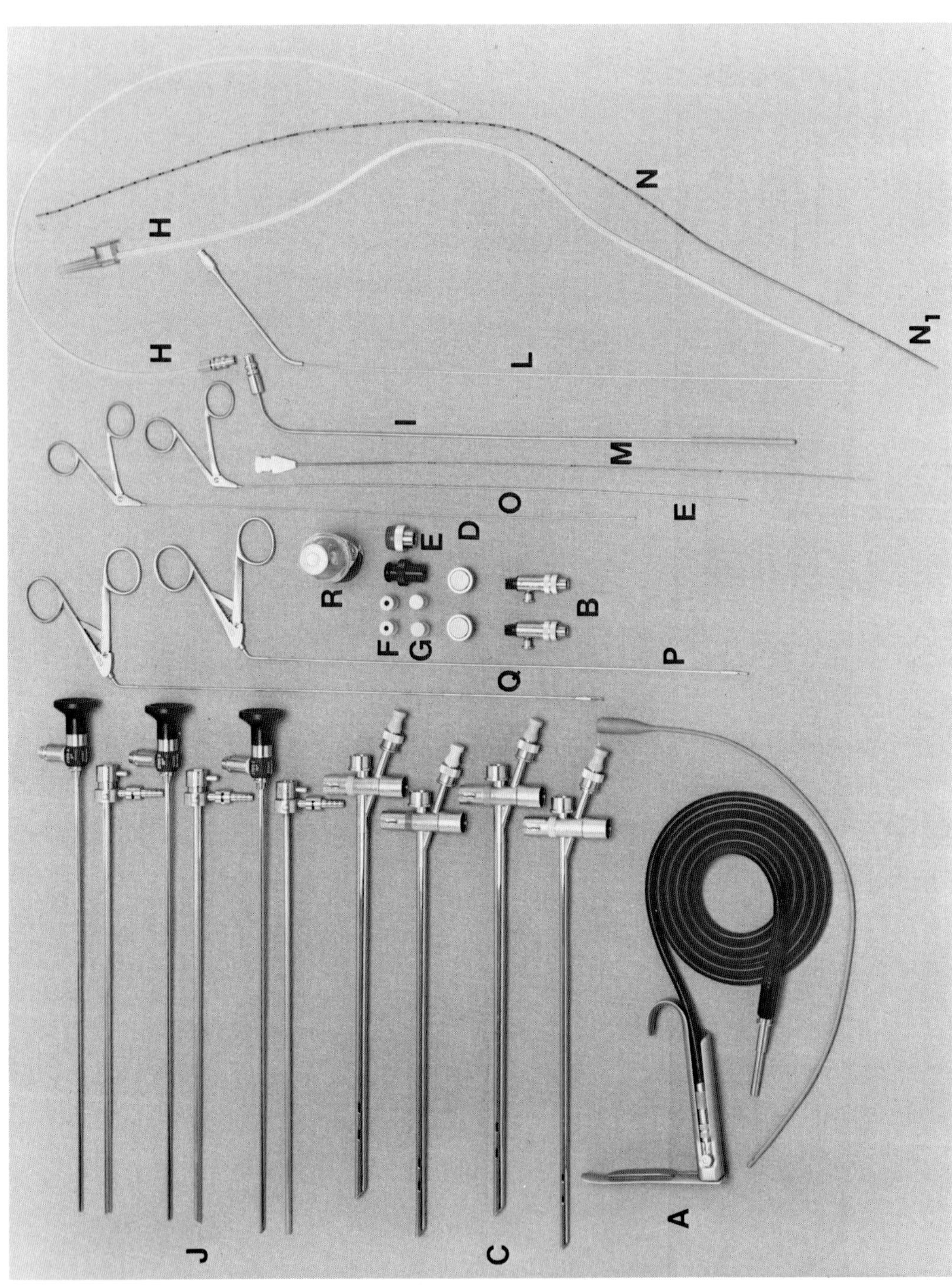
H
H
N
N_1
L
I
M
O
E
R
E
D
F
G
B
P
Q
J
C
A

Figure 4-4. *Instruments for use in intermediate-sized infants and children. (A) Laryngoscope with illumination and suction. (B) Prism light deflectors. (C) Bronchoscope sheaths: 3.5 mm × 30 cm; 4.0 mm × 30 cm; 5.0 mm × 30 cm; 6.0 mm × 30 cm; 3.0 mm × 26 cm; 3.5 mm × 26 cm; and 4.0 mm × 26 cm (not illustrated). (D) Glass windows. (E) Anesthesia or ventilator adaptor. (F) Nipples with holes. (G) Nipples without holes. (H) Two suction catheters, plastic, one to fit instrument channel and a larger one to pass through sheath. (I) Straight metal suction tubes (two), one with curved rubber tip and one with a velvet tip. (J) Storz Hopkins lens telescopes: 0°, 30°, and 70°, each with antifog tube and a telescopic bridge adaptor (not illustrated) for use when antifog tube is not used. (K) Telescopes for 26 cm bronchoscope sheaths (not illustrated). (L) Long injection needle. (M) Fogarty catheter. (N) Ureteral catheter. (N_1) Wire stylet for ureteral catheter for use in electrocoagulation (not illustrated; see Figure 5-3). (O) Biopsy forceps. (P) Alligator forceps. (Q) Peanut forceps. (R) Ultrastop.*

Method

Preliminary Investigation

Needless to say, all of the usual historical, physical, and laboratory studies will have been done, and special procedures, depending on the problem at hand, will have been performed and evaluated. Roentgenograms, scans, and any other helpful visual media should be at hand in the operating theater and in view on proper viewing apparatus.

Environment and Personnel

Bronchoscopy in infants and children is most effectively and safely performed in the operating room. Advantages include adequate space, availability of accessory equipment (optimally including x-ray capability), sterile technique, and, most of all, trained personnel for assisting in the procedure and, also importantly, in the event of difficulty or complications.

The team should include an anesthesiologist, an experienced head holder, a "scrub nurse" (a trained endoscopy technician), and a circulating nurse. It is also helpful and instructive for an endoscopic assistant or trainee to be present; in addition, particularly in the case of a neonate or ill child, a neonatologist or pediatrician is an important supportive member of the team. Such nonsurgical physicians can also profit a great deal by having the opportunity to directly visualize organs and pathologic conditions they are called upon to treat (Figure 4–5).

For most bronchoscopy in infants and children it is not necessary to have a special table with a fully mobile head rest. The standard table with the usual vertically moving headpiece is entirely adequate. A most important member of the team is a reliable and sensitive head holder, who moves and follows every manipulation of the endoscopist. A semisoft support lifting the child's shoulders and a temporary pillow for the head are the only props necessary.

It should be possible to control the room temperature. In addition to the respiratory, cardiac, blood pressure, and temperature monitoring by the anesthesiologist, rapid and repeated blood gas determinations should be available as needed.

Anesthesia

With modern improvements in anesthetic methods and in the experience of pediatric anesthesiologists, and with the availability of instruments with adequate airway space within the bronchoscope sheath, ventilation can be controlled precisely in a closed system incorporated in the design of the instrument. General anesthesia thus becomes the technique of choice for infants and children. This permits an unhurried, safe, thorough, and complete procedure to be done with a minimum of psychological trauma to patient and surgeon alike.

Introducing the Bronchoscope

With the shoulders propped up and a pillow under the patient's head, with a secure intravenous running, and with monitors in use, the infant is anesthetized as for laryngoscopy. The patient's head and body are draped with sterile material, and the

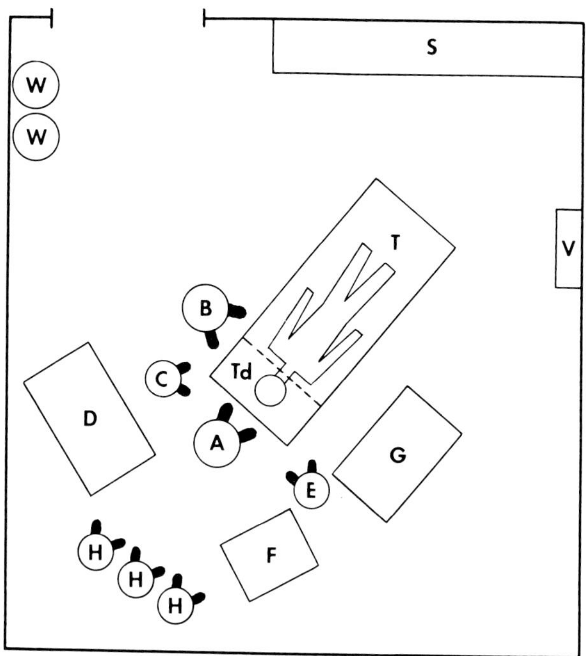

Figure 4-5. *Environment and personnel for bronchoscopy. (A) Endoscopist, standing or seated. (B) Head holder, seated. (C) Anesthesiologist. (D) Anesthesia equipment. (E) "Scrub nurse" (endoscopy technician) (F) Light source, air blower, and suction device. (G) Sterile instrument table. (H) Assistant, neonatologist, observer, student, etc. (S) Supplies and storage. (T) Operating table. (Td) Drop-off end of table. (V) X-ray view box. (W) Waste cans.*

surgeon, scrub nurse, and assistant use sterile gown and gloves. All instruments to be inserted into the airway should be sterile.

The usual proper position of the patient is described as flexion of the head and neck on the anterior chest, with subsequent moderate hyperextension of the head on the forwardly flexed neck. This seems more appropriate for the adult or older child. The neonate and infant bodies are so much more flexible and soft that we have found that *gentleness* in manipulation and instrumentation, with a proficient head holder, provides all the exposure necessary without unusual postures.

The gums or teeth are protected by a soft, moist sponge and the laryngoscope is inserted from the right of midline with the tip just at the base of the tongue pointed toward the suprasternal notch. A forward, lifting motion against the base of the tongue may expose the vocal cords by displacing the tongue to the left and elevating the epiglottis. At this point the bronchoscope may be introduced. A common error is insertion of the blade too deeply, resulting in airway obstruction from laryngeal occlusion and possible trauma to the epiglottis or upper larynx. The tip of the blade should be on the base of the tongue (Figure 4–6A) just proximal to the epiglottis. If forward elevation of the tongue at this point does not expose the vocal cords, the blade should be gently advanced slightly into the vallecula to elevate the epiglottis and expose the cords (Figure 4–6B). Again, too deep insertion has the opposite effect and will obstruct the airway and hide the cords.

The bronchoscope sheath selected should be small enough to pass through the glottis and subglottic area without causing trauma. Even the smallest sheaths afford

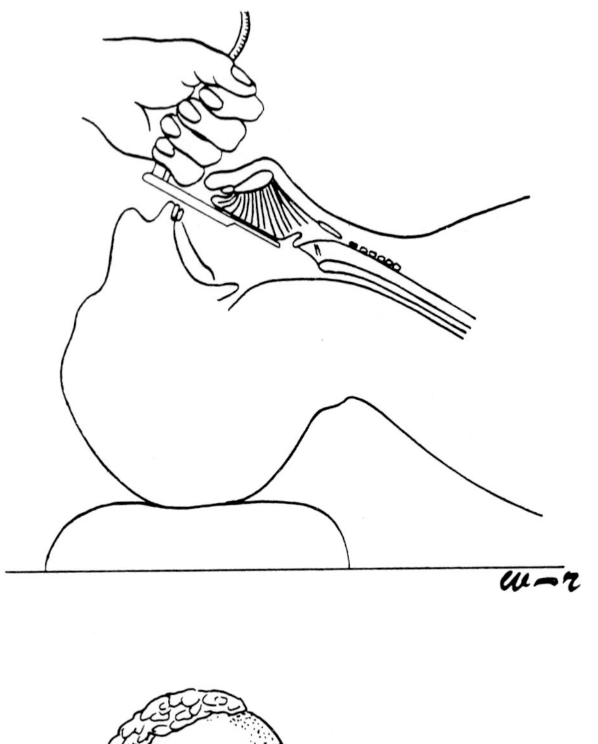

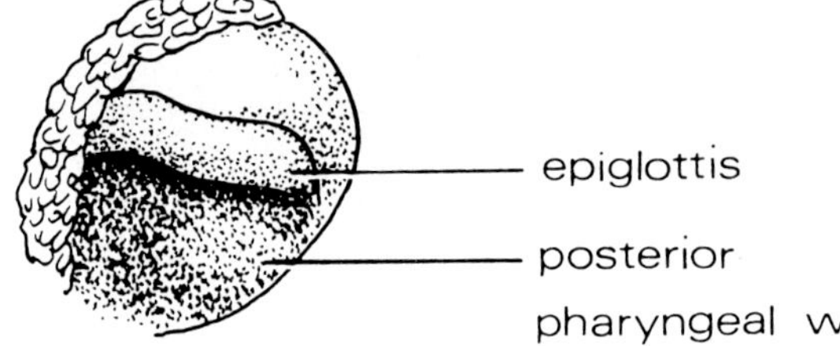

Figure 4-6A. *Method of introduction of bronchoscope. See text for details.*

excellent visibility because they all use the same telescope. However, the larger the sheath used, the greater is the space for ventilation and for manipulative procedures.

1. With the glottis exposed by the laryngoscope, the bronchoscope is held like a pencil in the right hand and passed carefully through the cords under direct external vision, using the lip of the bronchoscope, if necessary, to separate the cords.
2. An alternate method involves the use of the bronchoscope sheath with the telescope* already in place. With the bright and detailed view through the telescope, the epiglottis is located and tilted upward with the end of the bronchoscope, which is then passed through the vocal cords in direct view. The interior of the trachea is immediately verified (Figure 4–6C).

In method 1, using a proximal prism light, the passage into the trachea is verified (Figure 4–6C), a glass window is placed over the external orifice, and the instrument channel is blocked with a rubber nipple. In method 2, the telescope is removed and the end of the scope and the instrument channel are covered as above.

*"Telescope" means telescope and antifog sheath as a unit, when the antifog sheath is used.

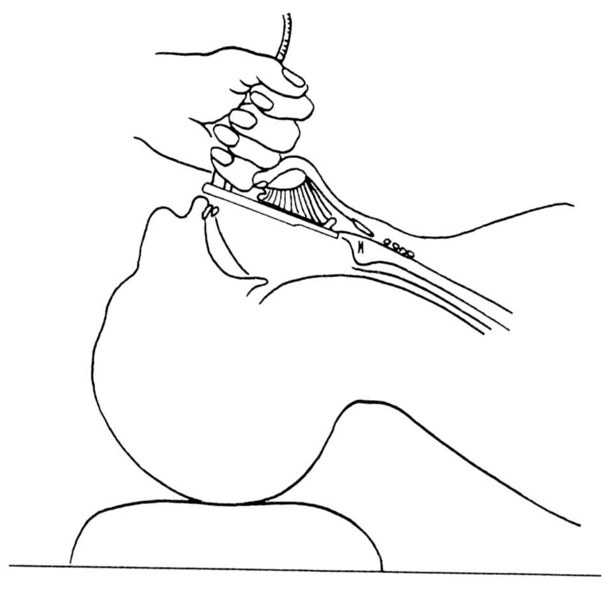

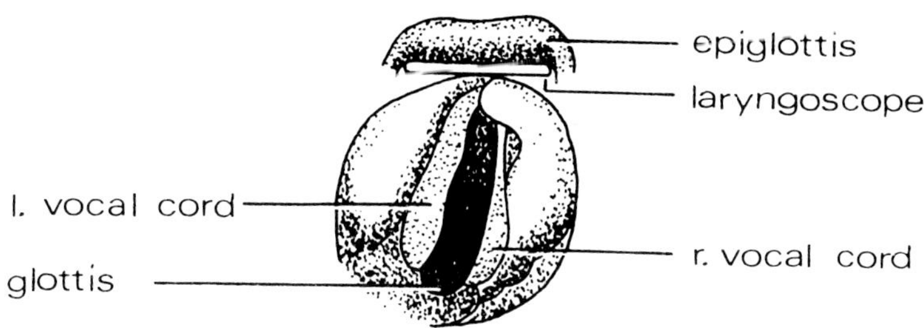

Figure 4-6B. *Method of introduction of bronchoscope. See text for details.*

After either method, the anesthesia adaptor is connected, and the anesthesiologist is given a large closed-circuit airway with which to ventilate and stabilize the patient if necessary. When the anesthesiologist is satisfied, the window is removed and the telescope* inserted. Examination of the tracheobronchial tree may now be carried out.

Suctioning may be carried out intermittently or continuously with a fine catheter passed through the instrument channel, saving time by maintaining a clear field during inspection. For more extensive suctioning with a larger catheter or tube, the telescope is removed and the suction tube is passed down the main channel of the sheath. Whenever a telescope is removed, the nurse dips the distal end in warm water and wipes it free of any foreign matter before handing it back for reintroduction.

Fogging of the tip of the telescope lens is very effectively prevented by use of the antifog sheaths used with the telescopes and connected with an air blower. Warming the telescope end in water prior to each insertion of the telescope is an addi-

*"Telescope" means telescope and antifog sheath as a unit, when the antifog sheath is used.

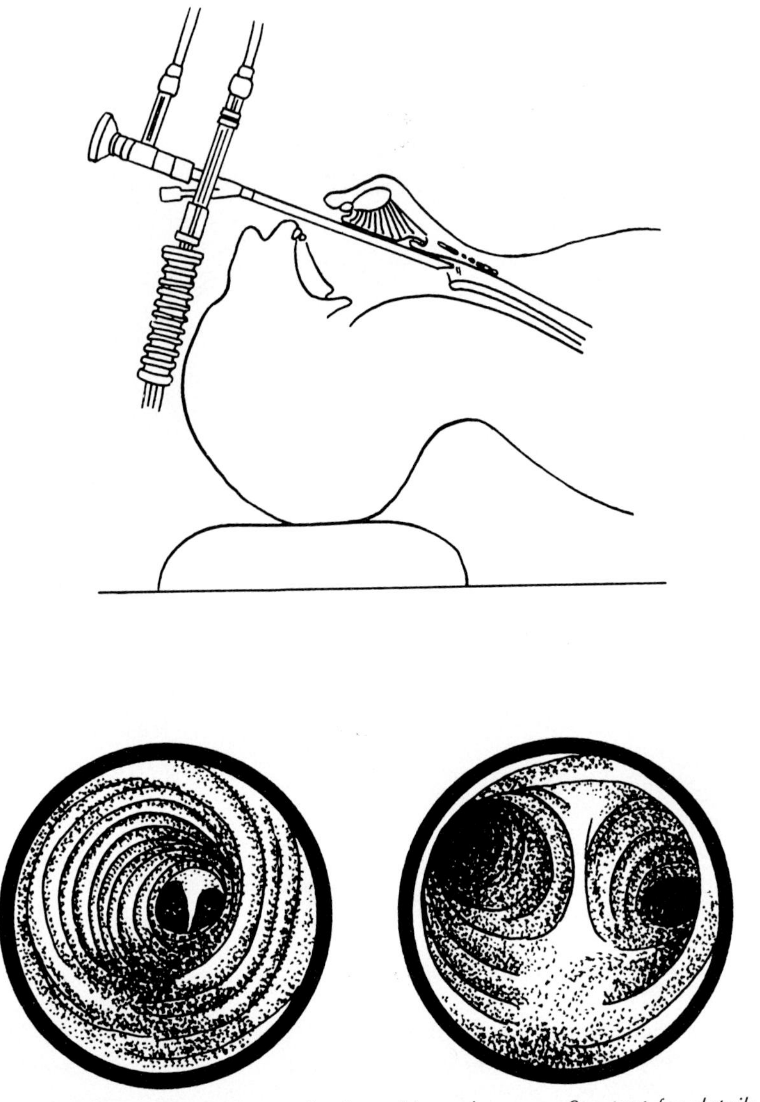

Figure 4-6C. *Method of introduction of bronchoscope. See text for details.*

tional aid. Sometimes it is necesssary or desirable to use a telescope without the antifog sheath. In such instances, warming the telescope end in water and the use of a drop of surface-tension-reducing solution (Ultrastop) at the end of the scope will also solve this problem.

Needles for injection or electrocoagulation (see Figure 5–3) can be passed through the instrument channel. Biopsy and foreign body forceps have been miniaturized so that they too can be introduced through the instrument channel and used in direct view of the telescope (Figure 4–7).

The instrument channel also accommodates small catheters for suction or instillation of solutions or for passage through a fistula. A Fogarty catheter is useful for the latter purpose, and its inflatable balloon can be used for temporary occlusion of the

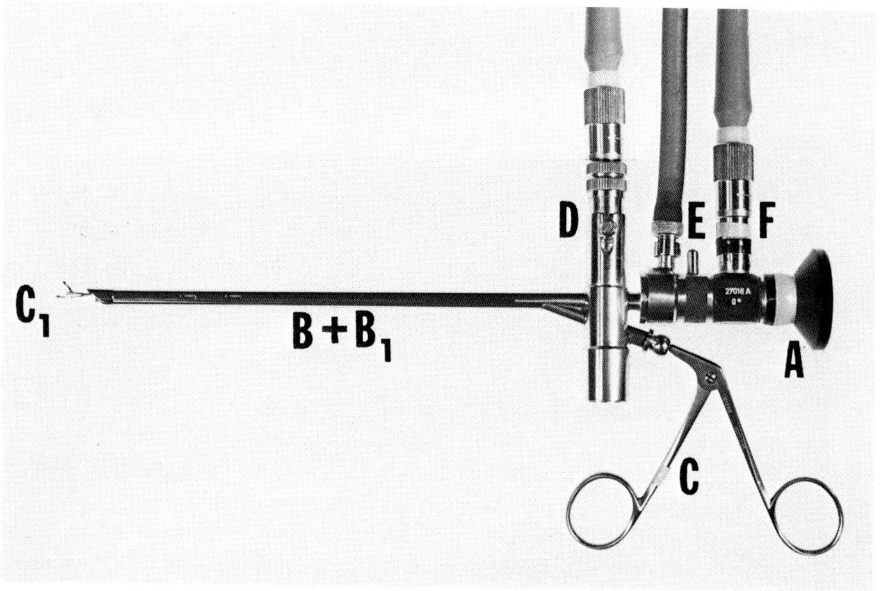

Figure 4-7. *Bronchoscope with foreign body forceps in front of telescope. (A) Telescope. (B + B_1) Bronchoscope sheath instrument channel. (C) Foreign body forceps handle with forceps in position in instrument channel. (C_1) Tip of foreign body forceps in open position in front of telescope. (D) Proximal prism light. (E) Antifog blower connected to antifog tube. (F) Fiber light connection to light-transmitting cable.*

fistula or for palpation during an operative procedure for fistula correction (see page 40).

Smooth instruments or catheters can also be passed alongside and outside of the sheath and still be used under direct vision of the telescope.

Removal of Foreign Bodies

Several hundred children die every year because of aspirated foreign bodies. The treatment of choice is the safe extraction of the foreign body with a bronchoscope. This is best done in a well-equipped endoscopic operating room, with a full and experienced team, and under general anesthesia by a competent anesthesiologist. The use of the open tube bronchoscope with its limited view and semiblind or blind groping attempts (the extracting instrument itself almost fills the lumen of the endoscope) often made this procedure hazardous, prolonged, traumatic, complicated, and even unsuccessful, leading to serious consequences and occasional open tracheobronchotomy. Telescopic tracheobronchoscopy has virtually put an end to these difficulties. Because of the clear, wide-angle view, even in scopes small enough to enter peripheral bronchial branches, the foreign body is quickly located. Under direct vision, the foreign body can be grasped with an appropriate extractor and removed (Figure 4–7). Some objects cannot be grasped because they are smooth and round or because they crush and fall apart (for example, a peanut). A slightly lubricated Fogarty catheter can usually be passed beyond such an object, the balloon somewhat inflated, and the foreign body and balloon withdrawn together.

Occasionally the view is obstructed by inflammation and/or edema. Sometimes this problem can be overcome by the direct local instillation of a topical vasoactive agent (such as diluted 0.25 Neo-synephrine), and sometimes accurate appraisal and evaluation will indicate discontinuing the procedure instead of prolonging traumatic manipulation, until conservative management may improve the tissue for a later attempt at bronchoscopic removal.[7]

In some instances combining endoscopy with fluoroscopy, with and without contrast media, is of help in locating and removing peripherally retained foreign bodies.[7]

Complications

Many of the potential complications associated with tracheobronchoscopy in infants and children are life-threatening. The forceful passage of a scope too large for the patient's airway, or any other traumatic passage of even the proper scope, may produce subsequent edema of the epiglottis, cords, or subglottic area with significant airway obstruction. Perforation of the trachea or bronchus is possible, with resulting pneumothorax or pneumomediastinum. The introduction of infection through poor technique and contaminated instruments can also have serious consequences. Finally, inadequate control of ventilation or partial mechanical obstruction of the airway during instrumentation can result in cerebral hypoxia and cardiac arrest. The possibility that any of these complications will occur in the hands of an experienced team has been measurably diminished by miniaturized equipment providing excellent visualization and maintaining secure control of ventilation.

References

1. Gans SL, Johnson RO: Diagnosis and surgical management of "H-Type" tracheoesophageal fistula in infants and children. J Pediatr Surg 12:233–236, 1977
2. Gans SL, Berci G: Inside tracheoesophageal fistual: new endoscopic approaches. J Pediatr Surg 8:205–211, 1973
3. Gdanietz, K: Personal communication.
4. Waag KL, Joppich I, Manegold BC: Endoscopic closure with Histoacryl of the recurrent oesophagotracheal fistula following oesophageal atresia. Z Kinderchir 17:24–28, 1975
5. Pompino HJ: Endosckopischer Verschluss Oesophago-Trachealar Fisteln. Presented at the Symposium on Pediatric Endoscopy sponsored by the Deutsche Gesellschaft für Chirurgie and the Deutsche Gesellschaft für Kinderchirurgie, Erlangen, West Germany, March 3–4, 1978
6. Gans SL, Berci G: Advances in endoscopy of infants and children. J Pediatr Surg 6:199–234, 1971
7. Hight DW, Phillipart AI, Hertzler JH: The treatment of retained peripheral foreign bodies in the pediatric airway. J Pediatr Surg 16:694–699, 1981

Esophagoscopy

CHAPTER 5

Stephen L. Gans

Endoscopy is quite indispensable for the management of many esophageal conditions, for it provides diagnostic information and methods of treatment unattainable in any other way. The origins and development of esophagoscopy have been described in Chapter 1 and, in a more detailed way, by H. D. Brown Kelly.[1]

Indications and Clinical Features

Dysphagia

Dysphagia is the most common indication for esophagoscopy in pediatrics and may be due to mechanical obstruction, neurogenic abnormalities, or pain.[2] Mechanical obstructions are either congenital or acquired and may be external to the esophagus as well as intrinsic.

Congenital stenosis may be a semilunar or diaphragmlike band or may consist of a short or long narrowed segment of the full thickness of the esophagus. Sometimes these problems are solved simply with dilatation, or the bands may be incised with electrocoagulation. Longer segments not responding to dilatation may require resection and anastomosis. In the lower third of the esophagus such stenosis must be differentiated from the stricture due to reflux esophagitis. Esophagoscopy may reveal inflammation or even ulcer formation, and biopsy of the mucosa is useful.

Acquired stenosis is either postoperative or the result of caustic or corrosive ingestion. Postoperative acquired stenosis is most often a complication of surgery for esophageal malformations and is usually managed by dilatation, with endoscopic diagnosis, direction, and supervision. Chemical burns of the esophagus are more accurately assessed and evaluated in both early and late phases by endoscopy, and dilatation, when necessary, is again monitored and supervised by direct observation (see Figures 16 and 17, p. v).

The diagnosis of *external obstructions* usually involves other modalities. Esophagoscopy may be useful for observing the internal effects of these conditions, such as inflammation, irritation, or infiltration, or for demonstrating localized compression or pulsation of a vascular ring.

Neurogenic or physiologic dysphagia is usually related to incoordination of the swallowing mechanism, and the role of endoscopy is to rule out mechanical obstruction or fistula, inasmuch as the symptoms may be the same. Achalasia, or cardiospasm, is generally considered to be a failure of coordination at the cardiac sphincter that results in a physiologic obstruction with proximal dilatation and hypertrophy of the esophagus. Treatment varies from simple esophagoscopic dilatation to forceful stretching with pneumatic or mechanical devices to esophagogastric surgery.

Pain may be due to foreign body impaction, cyst, tumor, cardiospasm, or esophagitis. All but the first of these conditions have already been mentioned. Problems relating to the removal of *foreign bodies* are related to the variety and differences in the quality and structure of the foreign body.

Fistula

The diagnosis of recurrent tracheoesophageal fistula or N-fistula (H-fistula) is best made by bronchoscopy (see p. 40), during which the opening can be seen with great clarity and even cannulated.[3] The fistulous opening may also be seen in the esophagus, particularly after flattening any folds by inflation. If there is any doubt, methylene blue can be dropped at the suspected site in the trachea and then quickly spotted by endoscopy of the esophagus. Other types of fistulas may also be detected by inflating the esophagus or manipulating its folds.

Gastroesophageal Reflux

A special word should be said about the diagnosis and management of gastroesophageal reflux. Esophagoscopy can demonstrate gastroesophageal sphincter incompetence in many instances, but other tests and modalities are more accurate for evaluating this abnormality. The main advantage of esophagoscopy lies in the demonstration of one of the serious complications of this condition, namely esophagitis. Early changes may be detected only by mucosal biopsy. As the lesion progresses, however, inspection reveals a reddened blush progressing to friability and bleeding on contact, dull granularity of the surface, and in severe cases frank mucosal ulceration and/or esophageal stenosis (see Figures 18 and 19, p. v).

Bleeding Lesions

Esophagoscopy is of considerable value in the diagnosis of upper gastrointestinal bleeding. It can rule out the esophagus as the site of bleeding, or it may demonstrate hiatus hernia, esophagitis or ulcer, esophageal varices (see Figure 11, p. v), or a bleeding tumor. It is also used as an alternative or supplementary treatment of esophageal varices by injection with sclerosing solutions.[4]

Equipment

Pediatric esophagoscopy has been enhanced by the development and availability of two types of esophagoscopes: rigid instruments with an optical lens system, and flexible fiberglass endoscopes that can be manipulated from the outside. Each has its advantages and disadvantages. The flexible scopes are equipped with suction, insufflation, and irrigating mechanisms that can be operated during continuous viewing. They have a greater degree of safety in less-experienced hands and can often be used without general anesthesia. They have almost no treatment possibilities, however, and the biopsy forceps usually provides fragments of mucosa that are difficult to interpret. Moreover, the clarity of the image is dependent upon the number of optical fibers contained in the cord—many fewer in the pediatric-sized scopes—and the view is much inferior to that obtained with the rigid telescopes. Finally, there is concern about the difficulties in sterilizing flexible endoscopes and the possibility of transmitting hepatitis.

The flexible scopes are essential for visualization of the stomach and duodenum and are superior for some diagnostic problems of the esophagus. These considerations are discussed in Chapter 6.

Equivalently sized rigid scopes have room for operating instruments for purposes of adequate biopsy, electrocoagulation, dilatation, foreign body removal, and injection in front of the clear, bright, wide-angle image provided by the telescope.

The reader is referred to Chapter 4 (p. 41) for information on illumination and antifog methods. It is also useful to have available laryngoscopes as previously described.

Table 5-1 provides a list of equipment for use in the neonate or small infant (see Figure 5-1).

Table 5-2 lists the setup for use in larger infants and in children (see Figure 5-2).

See Tables 4-1 and 4-2 for equipment and materials of general need in esophagoscopy.

Method

The reader is again referred to Chapter 4 (p. 48) for a detailed discussion of preliminary investigations and environment and personnel because they are the same for both esophagoscopy and bronchoscopy. I repeat only for emphasis the value of a reliable and sensitive head holder who moves and follows every manipulation and direction of the endoscopist, and of the assistance of an experienced endoscopy technician ("scrub nurse") who is completely familiar with the instruments and methods of preference of the endoscopist. The table and arrangement of equipment and personnel are shown in Figure 4-5. It must be possible to drop the head rest completely or to move the child's head over the end of the table in complete control of the head holder.

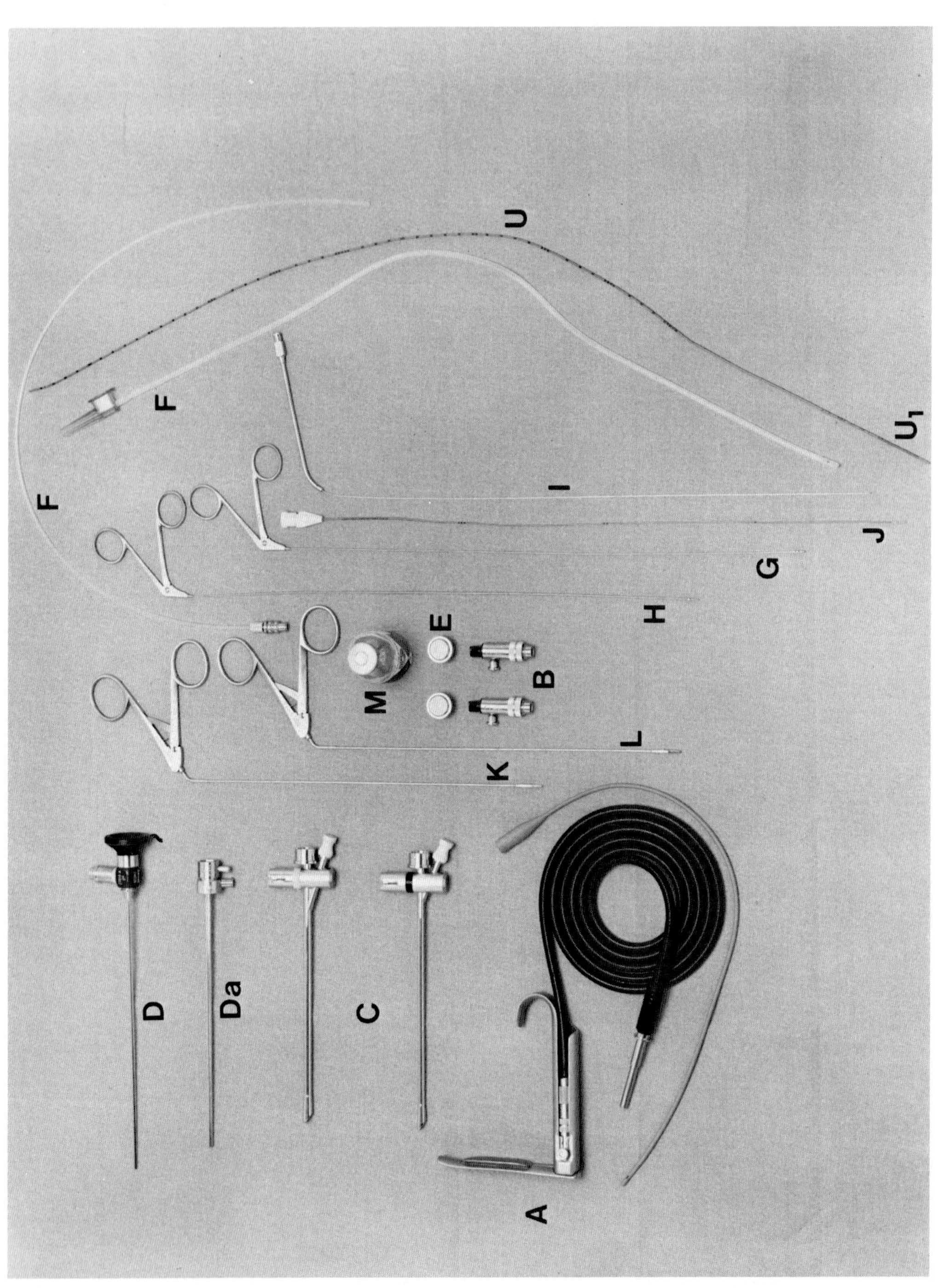
D
Da
C
A
K
L
M
B
E
H
G
J
I
F
F
U
U_1

Figure 5-1. *Equipment for use in neonatal esophagoscopy. See Table 5-1.*

Table 5-1

Equipment for Use in the Neonate (See Figure 5-1)

A.	Laryngoscope, suction and fiber light cable	
B.	Prism light deflectors	
C.	Esophagoscope sheaths (Storz), sizes 3 and 3.5 mm, length 20 cm	
D.	Storz (Hopkins lens) telescopes, 0°, with	
Da.	Antifog tube	
E.	Glass window plugs	
F.	Two suction catheters, plastic, one to fit instrument channel and a larger one to pass through the sheath, long enough to enter the stomach	
M.	Ultrastop	
G.	Biopsy forceps, 1 mm	For use through the instrument channel
H.	Alligator forceps, 1 mm	For use through the instrument channel
I.	Injection needle	For use through the instrument channel
J.	Fogarty balloon catheter	For use through the instrument channel
U.	Ureteral catheter	For use through the instrument channel
U_1.	Electrocoagulation wire tip*	For use through the instrument channel
K.	Alligator forceps	For use through the open tube
L.	Peanut forceps	For use through the open tube

*Not shown in Figure 5-1. See Figure 5-3.

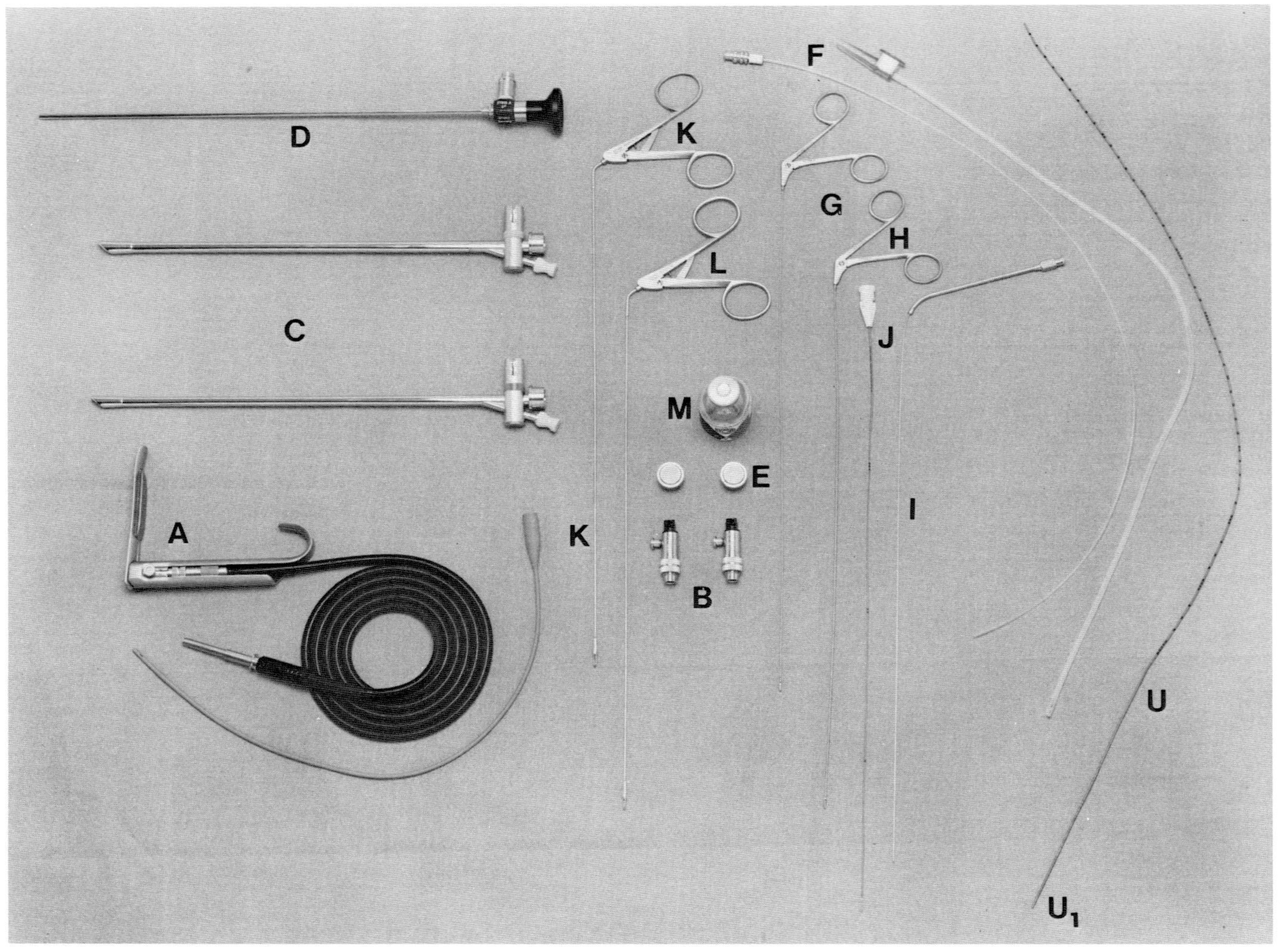

D
K
F
G
H
C
L
J
M
E
I
A
K
B
U
U_1

Figure 5-2. *Equipment for use in esophagoscopy of larger infants and children. See Table 5-2.*

Table 5-2
Equipment for Use in Larger Infants and Children (See Figure 5-2)

A.	Laryngoscope, suction and fiber light cable	
B.	Prism light deflectors	
C.	Esophagoscope sheaths (Storz), sizes 4, 5,* and 6 mm, length 30 cm	
D.	Storz (Hopkins lens) telescopes, 0°, with antifog tube*	
E.	Glass window plugs	
F.	Two suction catheters, plastic, one to fit instrument channel and a larger one to pass through the sheath, long enough to enter the stomach	
M.	Ultrastop	
G.	Biopsy forceps	For use through the instrument channel
H.	Alligator forceps	For use through the instrument channel
I.	Injection needle	For use through the instrument channel
J.	Fogarty balloon catheter	For use through the instrument channel
U.	Ureteral catheter	For use through the instrument channel
U_1.	Electrocoagulation wire tip†	For use through the instrument channel
K.	Peanut forceps	For use through the open tube
L.	Alligator forceps	For use through the open tube

*Not shown.
†Not shown in Figure 5-2. See Figure 5-3.

Anesthesia

In most instances, general anesthesia is preferred because it eliminates the need for cooperation usually required of a child and thus minimizes psychic trauma as well as instrumental trauma due to unexpected movements. The use of an endotracheal tube is an additional safety factor in preventing respiratory obstruction by pressure on the trachea by the instrument in the neighboring esophagus. Exceptions where one can forego the use of general anesthesia are the tiny neonate who can be well immobilized and controlled, the well-sedated or cooperative older child, or in some situations where the flexible scope is used.

Introducing the Esophagoscope

The patient is placed supine on the table with the shoulders propped by a sandbag or blanket roll and with the head completely mobile in the hands of the head holder.

The upper alveolar ridge or the upper teeth are retracted with the fingers of the left hand and the distal portion of the esophagoscope is grasped and controlled with the left thumb and forefinger. The proximal esophagoscope is manipulated with the right hand holding it as one would a pen and pencil. The tip of the scope is thus advanced along the right lateral border of the tongue and passed laterally to the epiglottis into the right piriform sinus. The larynx is lifted forward by the lip of the advancing esophagoscope to reveal the entrance of the esophagus. This may be clearly visualized after a few moments of observation, and the esophagoscope is then inserted into the cervical esophagus. If this anatomy is not quite clearly demonstrated, *very* gentle probing with the tip may reveal it and allow introduction of the scope. Another method of achieving exposure is with the use of the laryngoscope, taking great care not to obstruct the endotracheal tube or larynx. It must be remembered that the most common site of perforation occurring during esophagoscopy is the posterior portion of this field, and forceful manipulation is contraindicated.

If exposure and insertion cannot be accomplished with facility, the following method is a safe and useful alternative: A rubber or plastic catheter is passed through the esophagoscope and the cricopharyngeal sphincter, which forms this anatomic constriction, and then into the esophagus. The scope is then advanced over this "lumen finder" under direct vision, and as the esophagus is entered the guide is removed.

Inspection is carried out, keeping the lumen in view by manipulation of both the head and the scope. At the onset the head must be rotated posteriorly and adjusted as necessary. Manipulation of the instrument into the lower third of the esophagus is also facilitated by having an assistant straighten out the dorsal curve by placing his hands beneath the lower chest and elevating the dorsal spine. Occasionally difficulty is encountered in advancing the scope through the cardia and into the stomach. Again, this may be facilitated by first inserting a tube through the lumen of the scope and into the stomach, then gently passing the scope over it. The method and technique of examining the esophagus will of course vary with the problem being investigated and the pathologic condition expected.

Following diagnostic esophagoscopy, the patient is carefully advanced from clear liquids (watching for signs of perforation) to an appropriate diet.

Instrumental Manipulations

Biopsy

The use of the biopsy forceps through the instrument channel enables one to sample tissue in direct view of the telescope with careful inspection and selection of the most appropriate site or lesion.

Electrocoagulation

A 3 F ureteral catheter will pass through the instrument channel. A fine wire inserted through the lumen of this catheter will insulate it from the endoscope, and a protruding tip can be used for electrocoagulation if the proximal end makes contact with an electrocoagulating device. This capability can be used to cut congenital bands as well as for the usual indications for electrocoagulation. Care must be taken to keep both bare ends of the wire separated from the endoscope itself (Figure 5-3).

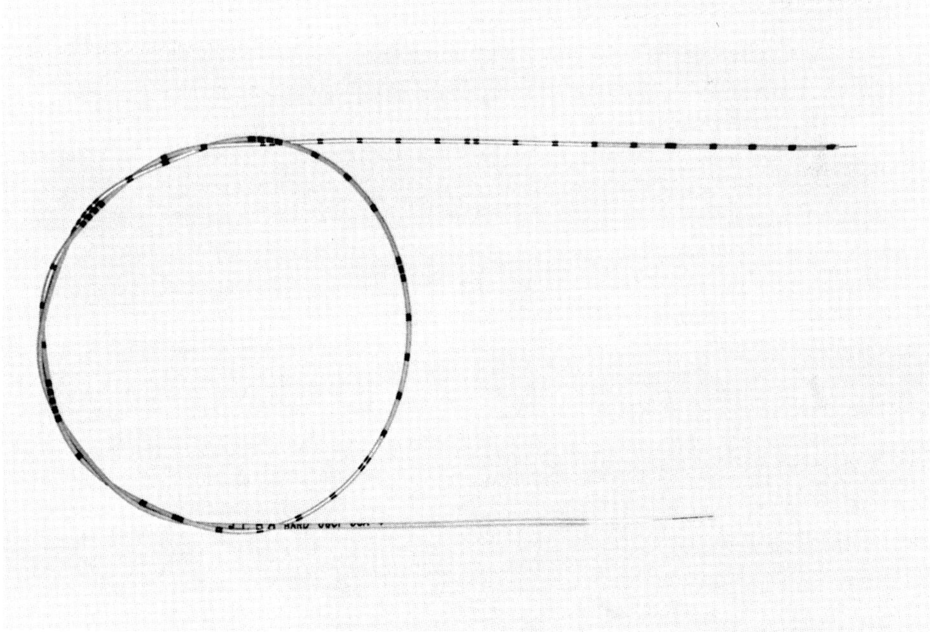

Figure 5-3. *A 3 F ureteral catheter will pass through the instrument channel. A fine wire inserted through the lumen of this catheter insulates it from the endoscope, and a protruding tip can be used for electrocoagulation if the proximal end makes contact with an electrocoagulation device. Care must be taken to keep both bare ends of the wire separated from the endoscope itself.*

Dilatation of Strictures

After visualization and evaluation of the stricture by esophagoscopy, a variety of methods can be used to initiate dilatation through the scope. A pinhole lumen may be identified and a small Fogarty balloon catheter passed through it. It is frequently possible to initiate dilatation by step-by-step inflation of the balloon, withdrawing it under direct vision through the stricture (Figure 5-4; Figure 13, p. v). When a gastrostomy is present, the Fogarty catheter can be passed into the stomach, where it is grasped and used to draw a string through the esophagus for subsequent retrograde dilatation with Tucker dilators. Esophagoscopy may alternatively be an aid in passing a string through a small orifice, for the same subsequent purpose. If there is any difficulty in removing the string or Fogarty catheter from the stomach, an endoscope can be introduced through the gastrostomy and the object grasped under direct vision by a biopsy or alligator forceps passed through the instrument channel.

Esophagoscopy is also useful to perform antegrade dilatation (see Figure 14, p. v). The scope is positioned flush with the stricture, the telescope removed, and then a tapered dilator is passed semiblindly or blindly through the stricture. This can be carried out only to the limits of the inside diameter of the tube. Therefore, either larger open tube conventional esophagoscopes can be used for larger dilators, because the procedure is "blind" anyway, or larger pointed rubber or mercury-weighted dilators can be used without a tube. Under any circumstances it is important to reintroduce the telescopic esophagoscope at the conclusion of these maneuvers, both to assess their effect on the stricture and to look for any serious complications such as perforation or bleeding.

Finally, it is possible to treat persistent strictures by direct-vision injection of steroids into the most appropriate areas, followed by dilatation[5] (see Figure 15, p. v).

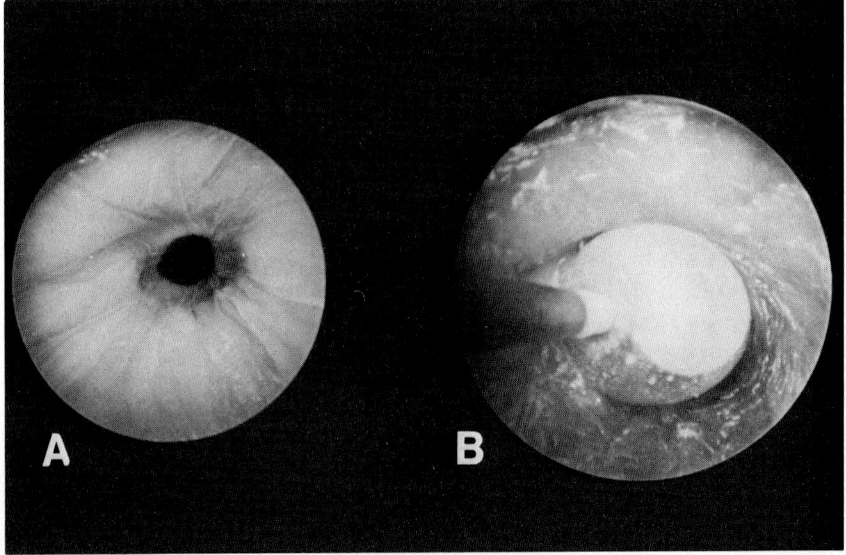

Figure 5-4. *(A) Esophageal stricture following repair of esophageal atresia. (B) Inflated Fogarty catheter emerging through stricture after dilating it. (From Gans SL, Berci G: Inside tracheoesophageal fistula: new endoscopic approaches. J Pediatr Surg 8:205–211, 1973. With permission.)*

Injection of Esophageal Varices

There are many reports of this procedure in adults and a few in children. Among them is a method described by Lilly[4] and used by us with modifications. A slotted esophagoscope enables one to accurately inject the varices with a special needle passed through the instrument channel and entering the scope a few millimeters short of the slot, which holds the varix in the lumen of the sheath, in direct view of the telescope (Figure 5-5A, B). Five percent sodium morrhuate, Sotra-dechol, or Sylnasol are used as sclerosing agents.

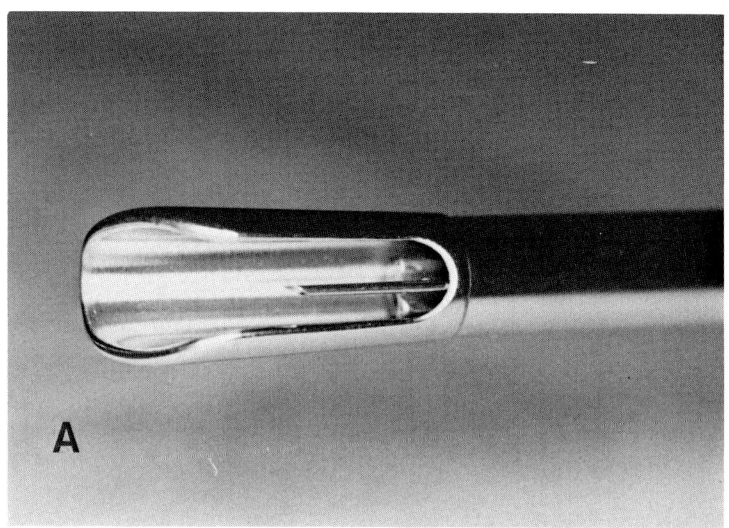

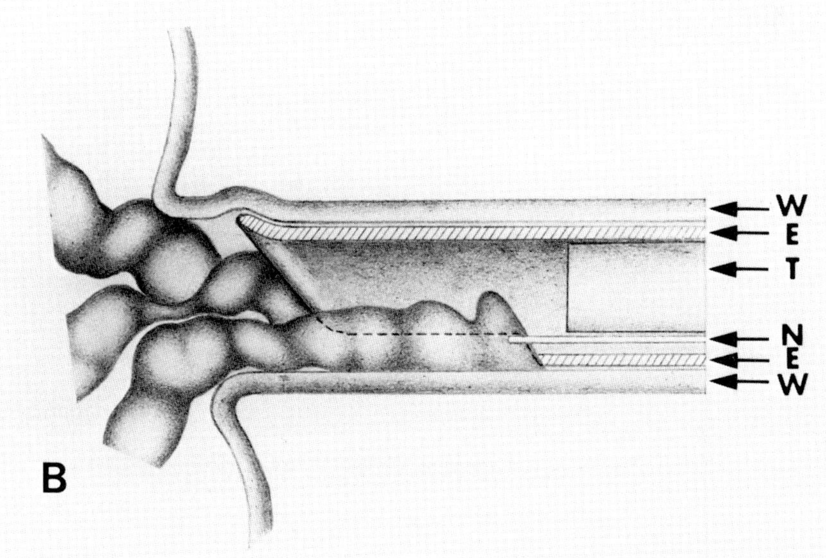

Figure 5-5. *(A) Illuminated end of special slotted esophagoscope with injection needle in place in front of the telescope. (B) Drawing of injection of esophageal varix: W, wall of esophagus; E, esophagoscope; T, telescope; N, needle in esophageal varix.*

It may be advantageous to compress the cardioesophageal junction with the inflated bag of a Foley or Sengstaken tube passed outside of the esophagoscope sheath, in order to prevent too rapid escape of the sclerosant from the varix. The scope itself is rotated after injection to compress the varix and the needle hole. One report[6] indicates that better results are obtained by injecting just outside of the lumen of the varix.

Removal of Foreign Bodies

When the hollow tube endoscope is used, the extracting instrument itself fills a good portion of the lumen necessary for viewing, and grasping is done in a semiblind manner. When the telescopic esophagoscope is used, the object can be located more quickly (see Figure 12, p. v) and less traumatically (no pushing), and a variety of grasping instruments can be used in full view of the telescope. It is important to be familiar and experienced with an assortment of instruments and methods. Hard and smooth objects may be difficult to grasp but may be successfully and quickly removed by directing a well-lubricated Fogarty catheter beyond the object, and, after slight inflation, drawing the catheter, object, and endoscope out together.

Some foreign bodies are more properly treated by carefully advancing them into the stomach, where they will usually pass spontaneously and safely through the intestinal tract.

Complications

Laceration and perforation are the greatest hazards of esophagoscopy but should be extremely rare in occurrence with examination alone. They may be more frequently associated with blind instrumentation, dilatation, or other operative maneuvers. We have observed no complications from esophagoscopy or associated manipulative procedures since we have been using the telescopic endoscopes. No doubt the incidence of these problems is reduced by better vision and by maneuvers carried out in full view.

References

1. Kelly HDB: Origins of oesophagology. Proc Soc Med 62:781–786, 1969
2. Gans SL, Berci G: Advances in endoscopy of infants and children. J Pediatr Surg 6:199–234, 1971
3. Gans SL, Berci G: Inside tracheoesophageal fistula: new endoscopic approaches. J Pediatr Surg 8:205–211, 1973
4. Lilly JR: Endoscopic sclerosis of esophageal varices in children. Surg Gynecol Obstet 152:513–514, 1981
5. Ashcraft KW, Holder TM, Leape LL: The treatment of patients with esophageal strictures by local steroid injection. J Pediatr Surg 4:646–653, 1969
6. Paquet KJ, Oberhammer E: Sclerotherapy of bleeding esophageal varices by means of endoscopy. Endoscopy 10:7–12, 1978

Fiberendoscopy of the Upper Gastrointestinal Tract

CHAPTER 6

Samy Cadranel
Pierre Rodesch

Following the adaptation of fiber optics for medical instruments, endoscopy of the gastrointestinal tract became, during the 1960s, a routine diagnostic and also therapeutic tool in most gastroenterology units in Japan, Europe, and America, and it is now used all over the world. Occasionally children were investigated in such endoscopic units,[1,2] but until recently, pediatric gastroenterology has been based on x-rays—black-and-white contrast images after a barium meal. During the 1970s direct visualization of the gastrointestinal lumen also became possible in childhood because of technical improvements of the instruments,[3] among which the reduction of the outer diameter of fiberscopes is the most important.

A few pediatric gastroenterologic units were interested in this new technique and started using it in children.[4–7] In most cases general anesthesia was used, at least in the beginning. Then, however, attempts were made to avoid general anesthesia[8,9]; and at present the use of general anesthesia versus sedation depends mainly on the availability of adequate instruments, the training of the endoscopist, and his experience in dealing with children.[10]

Our own experience, since 1971, is based upon more than 1000 examinations of the upper gastrointestinal tract in infants and in children from birth to 16 years. The use of miniaturized instruments, some of them prototypes,[3] allowed us to avoid general anesthesia in almost all cases. In our view fiberendoscopy in children should be a safe and painless routine procedure, challenging the predominance of the barium meal as a diagnostic tool in many indications in which x-ray studies are notoriously deficient.[11]

About 90 percent of the examinations in our series were performed for diagnostic purposes, including ERCP (endoscopic retrograde cholangiopancreatography); the remaining 10 percent were operative examinations, performed for such therapeutic indications as foreign body extraction, which can often be done under sedation, and esophageal dilatation, which is painful and requires general anesthesia.

Radiology and endoscopy are complementary techniques and probably will remain so for a long time.[8] X-ray study gives a better understanding of the topographic relationship of the organs and is generally performed under almost physiologic conditions without any preparation except fasting; it gives, however, a relatively poor view of the mucosal lesions. A closer view of mucosal details can be obtained by the double-contrast technique, but the procedure is no longer performed under physiologic conditions because of the use of relaxant drugs. It remains inferior to endoscopy for visualization of the mucosal lesions, and besides, with endoscopy easy immediate guided biopsies of lesions or suggestive areas can be obtained. Plain radiology is undoubtedly less invasive than endoscopy (if one does not consider irradiation, especially in infancy). As to the double-contrast technique, one should bear in mind that injection of drugs and intubation of the stomach or the duodenum are experienced by the small child as an aggression almost equal to passing a miniaturized gastroscope, providing that comforting psychological conditions and gentle handling of the child in a pleasant environment have been attended to.

Instrumentation

In the early 1970s the curiosity of a few pediatric gastroenterologists and surgeons was stimulated by the growing interest in endoscopy and its diagnostic success in adult gastroenterology. At that time, only the first generation of conventional fiberscopes were available, and as their diameter was large, only older children could be investigated, usually under general anesthesia. For smaller children and infants some investigators used the bronchofiberscopes, but these instruments were not designed for the examination of the alimentary canal and were thus poorly suited for pediatric endoscopic gastroenterology.[12]

The first pediatric fiberscope for gastroenterology was the Olympus PGF-S (pediatric gastrofiberscope) with lateral viewing and no biopsy channel, and it was soon abandoned. Then came the Olympus GIF-P (gastrointestinal fiberscope), an adaptation of the slimmest EF-P-A (esophagoscope), which, even with its limited two-directional bending, was very useful in infants because of its small outer diameter. A few years later came the four-way bending pediatric fiberscopes such as the Olympus GIF-P2, the ACMI TX-7, and, more recently, equivalent models by Mashida, Fuji, and Pentax (see Table 6-1). None of these instruments, however, is especially

Table 6-1
Synoptic View of Pediatric Fiberscopes

Instrument Make and Type	Outer Diameter (O.D.) (mm)	Tip Control	Bending Angle, Up–Down	Bending Angle, Left–Right	Field of View	Length of Bending Section (mm)	Biopsy Forceps	Electric Isolation	Optical Quality	Flexibility	Handiness
Olympus BF-B3R	5.3	2-way	160° 130°		80°	45	5 Fr	none	±		*
Olympus GIF-P	7.2 (6.8)	2-way	150° 150°		65°	80	5 Fr	none	±		+
Olympus GIF-P2	9.2 (8.8)	4-way	180° 60°	100° 100°	85°	65	5 Fr	+	+	±	+
Olympus GIF-P3	9.0 (8.8)	4-way	210° 90°	100° 100°	100°	65	5 Fr	+	++	+	+
Olympus JF-B3	11	4-way	130° 120°	90° 90°	64° side	58	5 Fr	+	++	+	+
ACMI FX-7	10.5 (9.5)	4-way	270° 270°	270° 270°	60°	60	7 Fr	+	±	±	±
ACMI TX-7	10.5 (9.5)	4-way	270° 270°	270° 270°	60°	60	7 Fr	+	±	±	±
FUJI UGI-FP	9.5 (9.5)	4-way	190° 160°	90° 90°	105°		7 Fr	+	+	+	+
MASHIDA FGI-SD	9.3	4-way	180° 90°	110° 110°	85°	?	7 Fr	+	+	+	±
PENTAX FG-18A	9.5	4-way	180° 80°	100° 100°	80°	?	7 Fr	+	?	?	+

*A special pushbutton device has been designed that can be adapted to the bronchofiberscope (only aspiration and air insufflation but no washing of the lens).

designed for pediatric endoscopy; they are actually slim instruments currently used as routine first-choice upper gastrointestinal fiberscopes for adults. An effort by the instrument makers to design truly pediatric fiberscopes would be most welcome, even if there are some commercial difficulties because of market size.

Let us now consider the characteristics of these miniaturized models (see Table 6-1). The main adaptation of conventional fiberscopes for pediatric use is the reduction of the diameter of the shaft, but this means that in very thin instruments two bending directions have been sacrificed (with only two left) or, in the larger ones, the caliber of the biopsy channel, which is also used for aspiration, has been reduced.

Outer diameter. Considering the tracheal compression hazards, the diameter of the fiberscope should not exceed 6–7 mm (or ideally 5–6 mm) in newborns and young infants. In older infants and in children, 8–9 mm can be tolerated, but, obviously, the smaller size is better accepted by the patient.

The *bending tip.* At present, technical limitations are such that it is very difficult to design a four-directional bending section in an instrument with a diameter of less than 8 mm. Therefore, in thinner instruments the tip can only bend in two directions. The *bending angle* should reach 180° in at least one direction (but perferably in two); asymmetry of the bending angles, usually encountered in almost all pediatric models available, is not a real handicap for an experienced endoscopist (Figure 6-1). The *length* of the bending tip is a very important feature. Excessive length is not adaptable to such small dimensions as the narrow curves in an infant's stomach (some areas cannot be explored properly and remain blind, such as the lesser curvature and some parts of the duodenal bulb); on the contrary, a bending segment that is too short is difficult to pass along the natural curves of the greater curvature of the stomach. The ideal compromise would be a 4–5-cm length for the bending tip.

Optical characteristics. The sharpness of the image is directly related to the quality and also to the number of fibers, which is necessarily reduced in pediatric instruments because of the reduction of caliber. However, the quality of the fibers equipping second- and third-generation fiberscopes has been very much improved and gives a very satisfactory image resolution. At the same time, the view angle has been widened from 65° to 90° and even 105°. The widening of the view angle un-

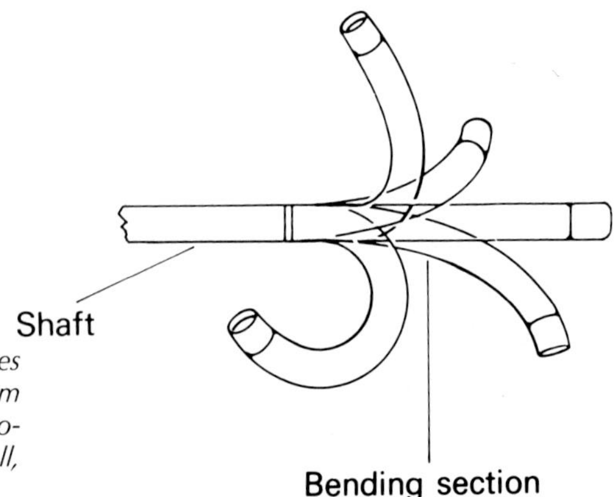

Figure 6-1. *Many pediatric fiberscopes have an asymmetrical bending tip. (From Cotton PB, Williams CB: Practical Gastrointestinal Endoscopy. Oxford, Blackwell, 1980. With permission.)*

doubtedly facilitates orientation and progression but requires a closer view of the mucosa for evaluation of details.

Flexibility of the fiberscope is also an important factor for the comfort of the patient; therefore, efforts should be made by the manufacturers to enhance flexibility in all pediatric models, especially the thinnest ones used in infants (Figure 6-2).

Aspiration, insufflation, and washing of the lens are essential in gastrointestinal endoscopy and automatic pushbutton systems are now widely used in all models (whether they are mechanically or electronically controlled makes little difference to the endoscopist but may be important in the maintenance and repair of the fiberscope). As one uses the right hand for manipulation of the distal extremity, the head of the instrument should be designed with an easy one-handed grip and manipulation of the control knobs for aspiration, insufflation, and washing (Figure 6-3A, B).

Accessories. The biopsy channel is usually small in pediatric fiberscopes (1.7 mm), except in a few larger instruments. The aspiration channel being common to

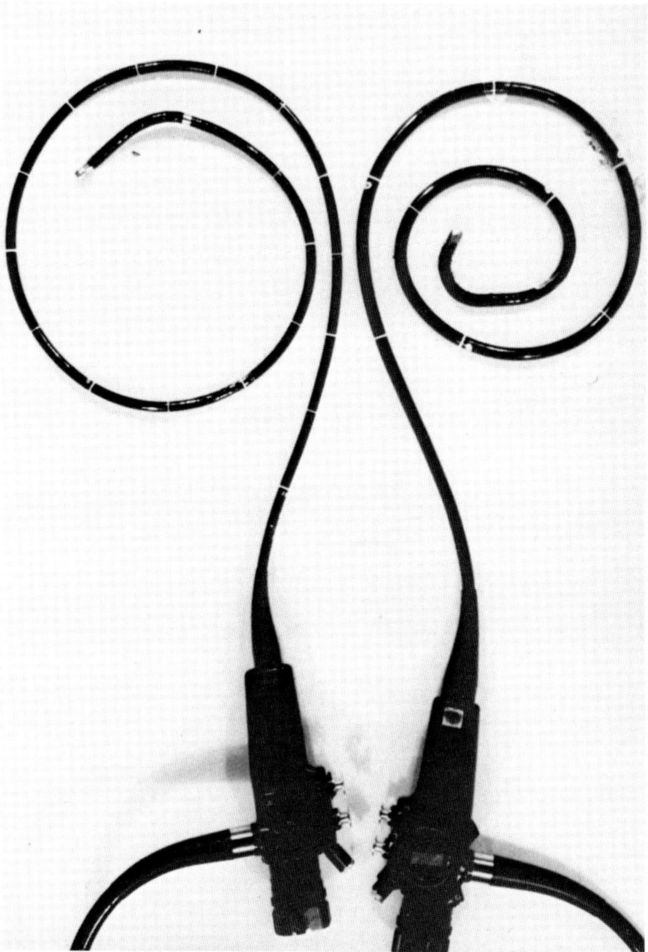

Figure 6-2. *Flexibility is an important factor; the four-directional 9 mm prototype is more flexible than the 7 mm GIF-P.*

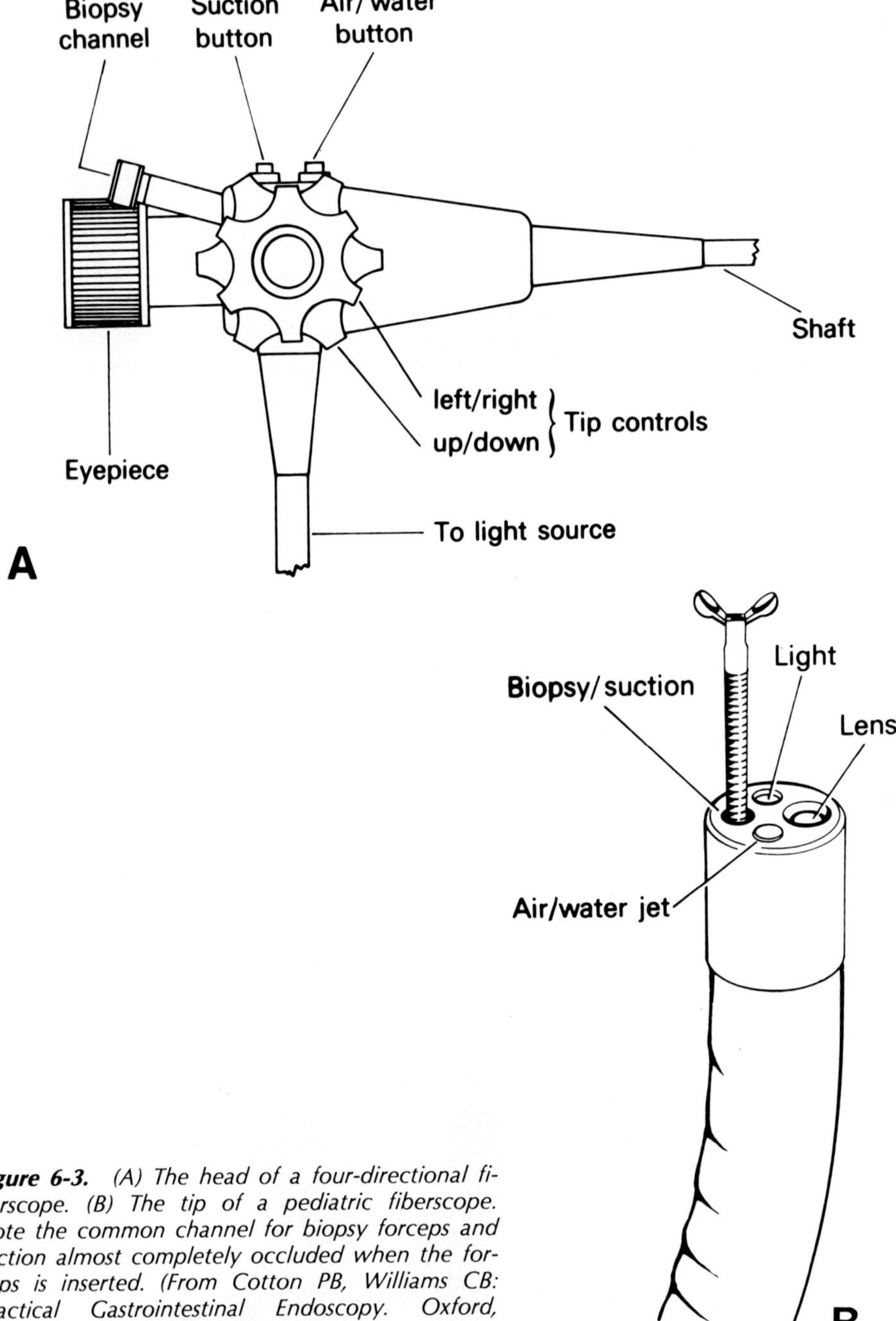

Figure 6-3. *(A) The head of a four-directional fiberscope. (B) The tip of a pediatric fiberscope. Note the common channel for biopsy forceps and suction almost completely occluded when the forceps is inserted. (From Cotton PB, Williams CB: Practical Gastrointestinal Endoscopy. Oxford, Blackwell, 1980. With permission.)*

the biopsy channel, aspiration is almost impossible when the biopsy forceps is inserted. One should be aware of this limitation and thoroughly aspirate the area before performing biopsies and also remember to aspirate the cavity between each biopsy. In addition, in some instruments the biopsy forceps passes with a great deal of friction through the channel when the fiberscope is bent and inserted into the duodenum.

Very recent models do obviate this handicap by slightly increasing the channel bore withuot changing the outer diameter (e.g., the Olympus GIF-P3), or even accepting a large biopsy forceps (2.3 mm) with only a slight increase in outer diameter (the ACMI FX-7). Each maker has its own accessories fitting the corresponding models of fiberscopes; among these are instruments designed for biopsy-taking, various shapes of foreign body removal forceps, diathermic loops, injectors, and the Eder-Puestow wire-guide dilator (Figure 6-4).

Sterilization and Maintenance

No complication has been reported in the literature concerning insufficient sterilization of the fiberscopes in pediatrics. This may be due to the relatively small number of examinations in pediatric compared to adult gastroenterology and also to the very rare indications for ERCP. The problem of sterilization, however, must be carefully monitored, as neglect of this important feature might lead to severe complications.[13]

After each examination, the external surface of the fiberscope is cleaned with soap and tap water, then soaked in a 0.5 percent chlorhexidine-alcohol solution, and then rinsed in a 0.02 percent chlorhexidine-water solution. The same sequence is applied for the biopsy channel, using the aspiration button. The biopsy–aspiration channel is further cleaned with a special channel brush. The water-feeding circuit is emptied after each examination. The biopsy forceps and other accessories must undergo the same treatment. The use of glutaraldehyde is probably safe but hypersensitivity could occur. The instrument should be cleaned and sterilized before the first use in a session to prevent bacterial growth during the storage period.

Lubrication of the accessories should be done before utilization using silicone preparations, and cleaning of the forceps jaws is important to prevent drying of residual material that in turn blocks normal action of the forceps.

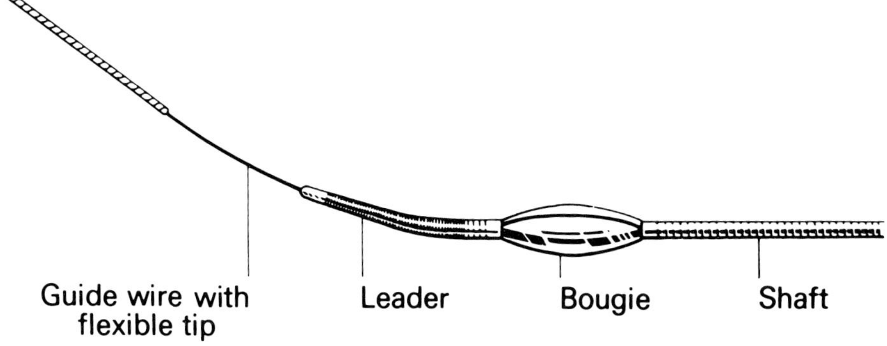

Figure 6-4. *Eder-Puestow metallic system for esophageal dilatations. (From Cotton PB, Williams CB: Practical Gastrointestinal Endoscopy. Oxford, Blackwell, 1980. With permission.)*

Careful cleaning is essential to prevent premature aging of the instrument through blockage of the different channels. The nurse and also the endoscopist should pay great attention to the cleaning and sterilization procedures, since contamination hazards to patients and also abusive and costly repairs can be avoided in so doing.

Preparation and Sedation

Using endoscopy as a routine diagnostic procedure means that it must be safe, gentle, psychologically acceptable by the patient and by his parents, and leave no bad memories. In our view general anesthesia must be restricted to painful or delicate examinations like esophageal dilatations, ERCP in small children, and extraction of certain oddly shaped foreign bodies.[14,15] For most diagnostic procedures sedation is sufficient. In newborns and infants light sedation (or even no sedation) with rectal Nembutal can be used. As apnea reflexes are possible in infants, it is advisable to stock in the endoscopy unit regularly checked resuscitation sets, including a readily available oxygen source, adapted masks, laryngoscope, several endotrocheal tubes, and the necessary material for starting a perfusion with antishock substances.

In children, the best results are obtained with pethidine (2 mg/kg body weight) together with atrophine sulfate (0.01 mg/kg). Diazepam, commonly used in adults, has rather disappointing results in children, whose cooperation cannot be relied upon with this type of sedation.

In older children a psychological approach is of utmost importance. Before the examination the patient is told all about it. Then, in presence of security-providing parents, whenever it is possible, the fiberscope is inserted in the esophagus and the child is allowed to follow his own examination with a teaching attachment, every maneuver being explained to the patient before and during the procedure.[16]

A fasting period of 6 hours prior to examination is necessary. In infants and small children, however, giving a bottle of water and sugar up to 1 hour before the endoscopy avoids dehydration and calms an otherwise overhungry, crying child.

The general setting of the endoscopy room plays an important role. The reception area must be cheerful and warm. The equipment and medical instruments may frighten or impress the child and therefore must be hidden or painted in light gay colors. Bright lights are not appropriate and should be dimmable. The child should be allowed to play with toys, and in general the decoration of the room must be adapted to the age of the patients, the general atmosphere resembling a kindergarten or a nursery rather than an operating theater.

Unless they are overanxious themselves, parents are allowed into the endoscopy unit and encouraged to reassure the patient. In our own experience, their presence usually calms the child and is an important factor of acceptance of the examination. A general atmosphere of kindness and minimalization of the procedure permits an undramatic endoscopy and, therefore, allows for a better follow-up examination when needed. The endoscopy nurse or assistant plays an important role, and she must be familiar with children and behave as maternally as possible.

The patient is placed in the left lateral position, with the head slightly extended. It is wise to keep the abdomen exposed, especially in infants, since there is a risk of excessive air insufflation; respiratory movements and color of the lips must be checked regularly. The way of holding the child differs according to the age of the patient. In toothless infants the mouthguard is unnecessary; the nurse supports the head and holds the arms loosely but firmly. The legs can move freely, which contributes to avoiding the impression of restraint. In older children (with teeth) the mouthguard is inserted first and must be carefully watched throughout the examination; the parents and the assistants hold the hands loosely but firmly. The different steps are explained to the child, who is invited, on several occasions to follow his own examination with the teaching attachment. It is not rare to observe infants fall asleep during the examination and teenagers follow their own investigation with enthusiastic attention.

Small children, unfortunately, cannot understand the situation and try to resist; a firm hold of arms and legs, together with larger doses of sedatives, is required.

Technique of Examination

The adult patient is generally aware of his problem and willing to undergo an examination. He is usually cooperative; therefore, the stress of hurry is not excessive and the endoscopist can afford to perform his examination without haste. Total cooperation of the pediatric patient is unusual and seldom sustained; therefore, the examination must be as comprehensive as possible in a very short time. This requires experience and gentleness by the endoscopist, with precise manipulation, no false maneuvers, and very good technique.

Before the first examination of a session and between each procedure, the instrument is rinsed in a disinfecting solution and checked, before insertion, for patency and effectiveness of channels and proper movement of the control wheels. The head of the instrument is held with the left hand, the three last fingers and the palm firmly holding the head and leaving the thumb free, so that it can be used to mobilize the "up" and "down" tip control wheel, and the second finger free to activate aspiration or air and water buttons. The tip of the instrument and its shaft are held with the right hand, in order to control pushing and pulling movements. As a general rule, the fiberscope is maneuvered by the endoscopist alone; the lateral movements are obtained either by rotating the whole instrument, the left hand controlling its head and the right one its shaft, or by using the corresponding control wheel, usually with the right hand, while the assistant holds the shaft of the instrument. Usually, movement of the whole fiberscope is used for advancing in the procedure, the use of the "left and right" control knob being reserved for the smaller and more delicate movements such as entering the pylorus or taking a biopsy. Most popular fiberscopes have an asymmetric bending tip (e.g., the Olympus GIF-P2): 180° up (sometimes more), 60° down, and 90° left and right (Figure 6-1). This implies that one uses the more efficient "up" position in almost all possible situations throughout the examination, varying its angulation following the natural curves of the alimentary canal and giving lateral angulation by moving the instrument sideways.

Introduction of the tip of the instrument into the mouth is usually easy, providing the child has been adequately prepared psychologically. First the mouthpiece is inserted between the anterior teeth, and then the tip of the instrument is inserted. Passage of the tip of the instrument is a very important step in the examination and must be done smoothly and in one motion because harmless, easy passage is followed by good acceptance and relaxation of the patient, whereas false movements can cause fear and resistance and thus greatly handicap the rest of the examination.

Under visual control the tip of the fiberscope, bent into the "up" position at 60°, follows the palate arch; when a swallowing movement occurs—this can be provoked by a small amount of water insufflated through the washing system—the instrument's tip is pushed into the esophagus while deflection of the tip is corrected back to the neutral position and actively maintained in this position by controlling the corresponding knob. By so doing one avoids a common error: when the tip of the instrument is left free, it is usually overbent into a U-turn position or pushed into the tracheal orifice.

Observation of the esophagus is preferably done during insertion rather than removal. The cardia should be examined carefully for competence, inflammatory changes, or herniation through the diaphragmatic ring.[17] The herniated pouch or an open cardia can also be investigated in the "retrovision" position from the gastric cavity (see Figure 20, p. v).

Passage into the stomach must be done with caution. At the edge of the gastric part of the cardia, rapid but careful insufflation of air is necessary to avoid traumatizing the posterior wall of the stomach. At this moment of the examination, with the child lying on his left side, the tip of the instrument is high in the body of the stomach, and one can see (Figure 6-5) the anterior wall corresponding to the "up" position, the posterior wall to the "down" one, the smooth lesser curvature to the "right," and the rugose greater curvature to the "left." The tip of the instrument is then advanced further on the body of the stomach, and examination of the cardia in retrovision is obtained by overaccentuating the "up" and "left" positions and gently withdrawing the shaft of the instrument for a closer view of the cardiac orifice (Figure 6-6).

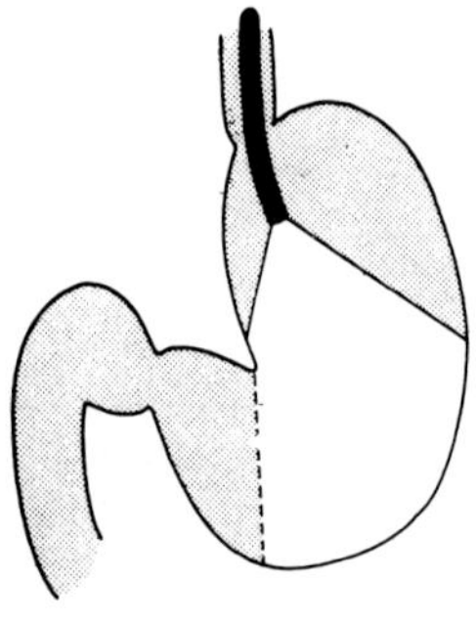

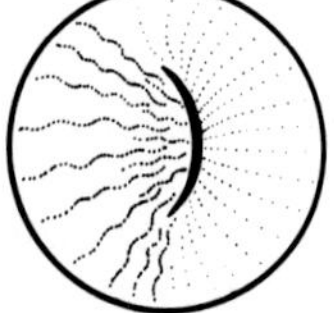

Figure 6-5. *Passage of the tip of the fiberscope through cardia (top); view from this position (bottom). See text for details. (From Cotton PB, Williams CB: Practical Gastrointestinal Endoscopy. Oxford, Blackwell, 1980. With permission.)*

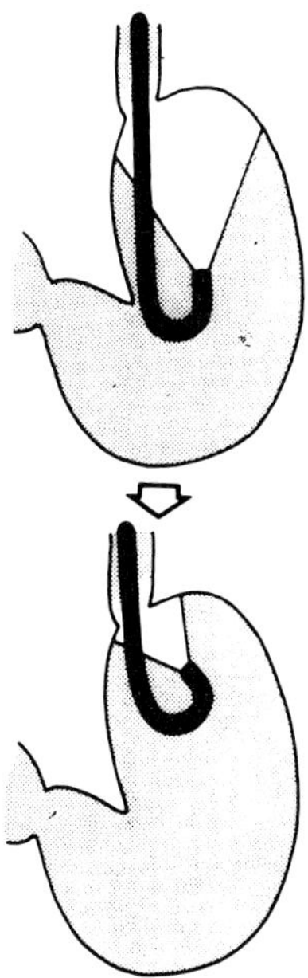

Figure 6-6. *Retrovision of the cardia. See text for details. (From Cotton PB, Williams CB: Practical Gastrointestinal Endoscopy. Oxford, Blackwell, 1980. With permission.)*

The control wheels are then turned back to neutral position and the instrument pushed in again gently on the body of the stomach, so that one can proceed to the examination of the angulus and enter the antrum, preferably by using the "up" position combined with a clockwise rotation of the whole instrument. By this movement the two hands operate in coordination and the advance can be accomplished in a single step; whereas to use the lateral control knob the operator's right hand must release the tip of the instrument, and the whole advancing movement needs an intermediate stop-and-watch step at the level of the angulus (Figures 6-7, 6-8).

Advancement to the pylorus is obtained by progressively reducing the "up" flexion position and advancing the instrument forward. When the pylorus is in view, a slight downward movement might be useful to pass it and enter the duodenal bulb; at this moment light insufflation of air together with moderate withdrawal of the tip are necessary to distend the bulb and to obtain a better view of its walls.

The superior duodenal angle appears sharply downward and to the right when considering the lens index. Thus it is rather difficult to examine the duodenum when using a pediatric instrument because of the weak 60° downward bending capacity. This difficulty can be obviated by carefully introducing the tip of the instrument beyond the duodenal angle; then, with the knobs back to the neutral position, the fiberscope is rotated from head to tip in a clockwise movement of 120° to 150° with the tip progressively bent to the "up" position as far as 150°. The characteristic ringed aspect of the duodenum is then visualized. Further progression of the tip of the instrument can be obtained by partial withdrawal of the shaft, thus unwinding the intragastric loop of the fiberscope, which results in a passive advancement of its tip into the second part of the duodenum (Figures 6-9, 6-10).

During all these maneuvers the shaft of the instrument between the patient's head and the endoscopist's right hand must be kept as straight as possible to aid orientation and ensure direct transmission of the rotatory movements.

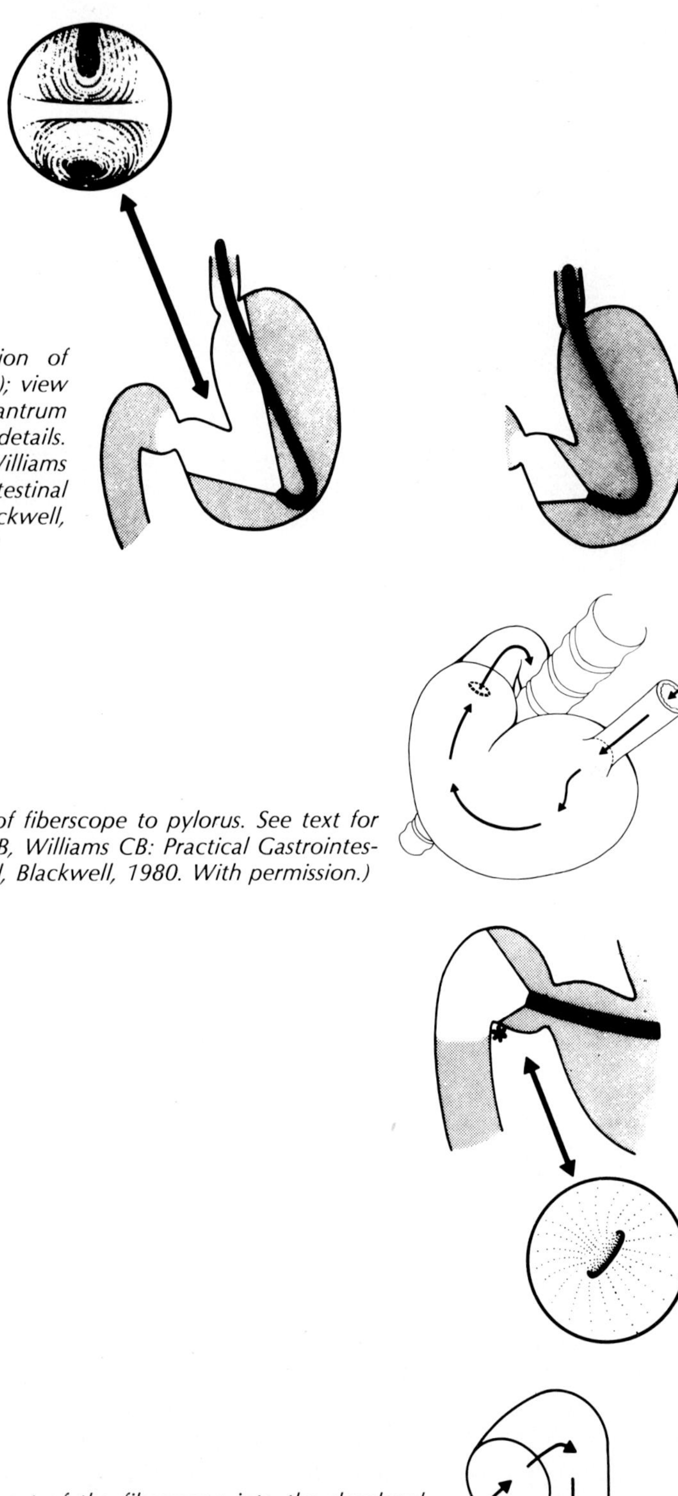

Figure 6-7. *Examination of the gastric angulus (left); view of pylorus from the antrum (right). See text for details. (From Cotton PB, Williams CB: Practical Gastrointestinal Endoscopy. Oxford, Blackwell, 1980. With permission.)*

Figure 6-8. *Insertion of fiberscope to pylorus. See text for details. (From Cotton PB, Williams CB: Practical Gastrointestinal Endoscopy. Oxford, Blackwell, 1980. With permission.)*

Figure 6-9. *Advancement of the fiberscope into the duodenal bulb (top) and progress through the superior duodenal angle (bottom). See text for details. (From Cotton PB, Williams CB: Practical Gastrointestinal Endoscopy. Oxford, Blackwell, 1980. With permission.)*

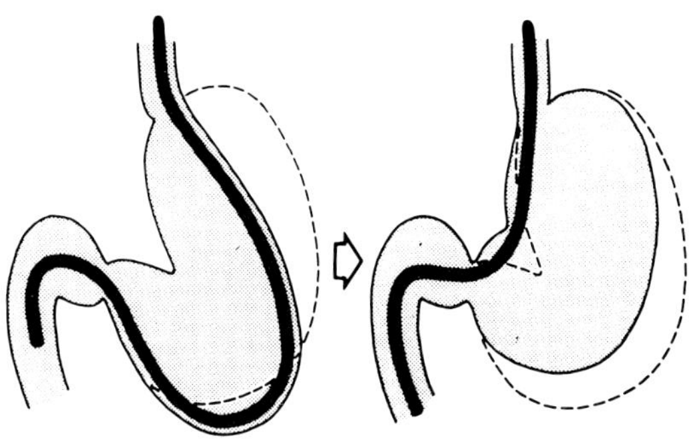

Figure 6-10. *Technique for progressing through the duodenum. See text for details. (From Cotton PB, Williams CB: Practical Gastrointestinal Endoscopy. Oxford, Blackwell, 1980. With permission.)*

Air insufflation must be minimal, especially in infants. Careful examination and topographic localization of all the lesions must precede biopsy sampling, as bleeding may obscure these lesions. Because of the narrow biopsy channel in most pediatric endoscopes, aspiration is inefficient once the biopsy forceps is inserted, and aspiration should be performed between two biopsy samples. Passing the biopsy forceps through the corresponding channel is not easy when the tip of the fiberscope is in a sharply bent position such as that used for entering the duodenum. Besides prophylactic lubrication of the forceps and the channel, it is sometimes necessary to pull the fiberscope back into the stomach, insert the biopsy forceps as far as the tip of the instrument, and then progress forward into the duodenum.

With the third-generation instruments this excessive friction of the biopsy forceps against the walls of the biopsy channel has been improved (Olympus GIF-P3, ACMI FX-7, Mashida, Pentax, and Fuji).

Indications

The main symptoms leading to a diagnostic endoscopy of the upper gastrointestinal tract in childhood are persistent vomiting, gastroesophageal reflux, abdominal pain, bleeding, ingestion of caustic products, and suspicion of portal hypertension; cholangiopancreatography is rarely indicated in childhood.[18,19] (See Table 6-2.)

Indications for therapeutic endoscopy are removal of foreign bodies, dilatation of esophageal strictures, and, rarely, polypectomy of gastric or duodenal polyps.

Diagnostic Endoscopy

Persistent vomiting is a frequent problem in infancy. The first investigative study is usually radiologic, showing the overall topography of the esophagus and the stomach and demonstrating reflux with or without a hiatal hernia.[11] Other studies include the Tuttle test, manometric recording of the lower esophageal sphincter (LES) pressure, long duration recording of the esophageal pH, and detection of the gastroesophageal reflux by scintiscanning. The place of fiberendoscopy is to demonstrate the result of longstanding repeated reflux of acid gastric juice on the lower esophageal mucosa; whereas mild or early esophagitis can be missed by roentgenologic studies, the reddening of the mucosa as seen through the fiberscope suggests esophagitis and guided biopsies confirm the diagnosis. Early detection of these le-

Table 6-2
Indications for Upper Gastrointestinal Fiberendoscopy

Diagnostic		Therapeutic	
Chronic vomiting	253	Esophageal dilatation	139
Abdominal pain	167	Injection of corticoids	15
Bleeding	73	Foreign bodies removal	59
Ingestion of corrosive products	66		
Portal hypertension	28		

Endoscopic Findings	
Cardial incompetence (reflux, hiatal hernia)	120
Esophagitis	103
Mallory-Weiss syndrome	10
Gastritis	52
Gastric or duodenal ulcers	45
Duodenitis	26
Hypertrophic pyloric stenosis	19
Rare lesions	10

sions and monitoring of the efficacy of the treatment is important for prevention of severe peptic esophagitis and its consequences: fibrosis, scarring, shortening, and stricture of the esophagus.

Abdominal pain, a very frequent complaint in childhood, often has a psychosomatic background and is seldom due to an organic cause. However, when pain is related to meals, is mainly located in the epigastrium, and is persistent, an endoscopic examination should be considered, even if a previous roentgenologic study is normal. The endoscopist should look for gastric or duodenal ulcerations, gastritis, or duodenitis.

Bleeding of the upper gastrointestinal tract can occur at any age but is more frequent in neonates, infants, and teenagers.[20] The diagnostic findings include esophagitis, bleeding varices, Mallory-Weiss syndrome, acute gastritis and duodenitis, peptic ulcer of the stomach or the duodenum, coagulopathies, angiomata, polyposis, and gastric or duodenal lymphoma.

Since most of these lesions are of the superficial mucosa, x-ray studies are frequently not diagnostic, particularly in the acute phase when the stomach is full of blood. Fiberendoscopy performed soon after the acute bleed (within 24 hours) has a high diagnostic accuracy. Sometimes the procedure must be repeated after careful washing of the stomach. Multiple lesions are not rare, and determining the primary cause of the bleeding may sometimes be difficult.[21]

Esophageal varices are more accurately detected by endoscopy than by any other technique. It is also possible to evaluate their severity and follow their progress after therapy. Therefore, systematic endoscopy is indicated in all cases of suspected portal hypertension, such as in cirrhosis, portal vein cavernomas, Budd-Chiari syndrome, and unexplained splenic enlargement.

Caustic esophagitis. Most often doubt is raised as to whether the offending agent has really been swallowed by the child. An early endoscopy is very useful in order to confirm caustic lesions of the esophagus and to evaluate their severity and only then undertake energic supportive measures that are superfluous when no lesion has been found.[15]

ERCP (endoscopic retrograde cholangiopancreatography) is rarely performed in children because the instruments are too large and the indications are uncommon.[18] In older children, mainly teenagers, occasional indications are chronic pancreatitis, choledochal cyst, and other biliary tract diseases (see Chapter 7).

Therapeutic Endoscopy

Foreign body removal. Swallowing of foreign bodies is very frequent in childhood. Most often the foreign body progresses without difficulty and is eliminated by normal peristalsis.[2,22] In some instances, however, the foreign body remains immobilized in the esophagus and may be responsible for perforation and subsequent mediastinitis.

Frequently one is dealing with coins or round objects that can be pushed into the stomach when removal by use of a special miniaturized forceps is too difficult. In some cases, however, the use of a rigid endoscope is necessary, and then the examination requires general anesthesia (see Chapter 5). Most objects lying in the stomach are passed spontaneously unless their composition, being harmful to the mucosa, or their odd shape, posing difficulty for normal evacuation, indicates an endoscopic removal.

Dilatation of esophageal strictures. An alternative to classical bougienage with rubber bougies is the Eder-Puestow system (see Figure 14, p. v) in which a metallic wire is passed through the stenotic zone under endoscopic control; on this metallic guide, a dilator with progressively larger metallic olives is passed. Hollow rubber bougies can also act as dilators on the same guide. Metallic olives have been designed for pediatric use[14] (Figure 6-11). Stenoses may occur after operation for congenital esophageal atresia, in the distal esophagus following peptic reflux, following ingestion of caustic agents, or after exposure to radiotherapy (see Table 6-3).

Injection of corticoids (see Figure 15, p. v) or sclerosing compounds in the esophageal wall is possible with endoscopic injectors fitting the biopsy channel bore. Corticoids seem to reduce the scarring and fibrosis occurring after each dilatation for caustic esophagitis. The local corticoid is usually injected before the dilatation procedure.[15] Sclerosis of esophageal varices can be accomplished with the same type of injector and might be very helpful in bleeding varices as a palliative therapy (see Chapter 5).

Polypectomy is a rare indication in childhood because of the rarity of polyps in the stomach or duodenum (Peutz-Jeghers syndrome).[10] Polypectomy in the upper gastrointestinal tract is no different than colonic polypectomy (see Chapter 8).

Complications and Contraindications

No severe complications have been noted in our series. Except for the infrequent side-effect of vomiting due to the premedication, the examination is well tolerated. In infants one must be aware of vagal reflexes occurring with overinsufflation of air,

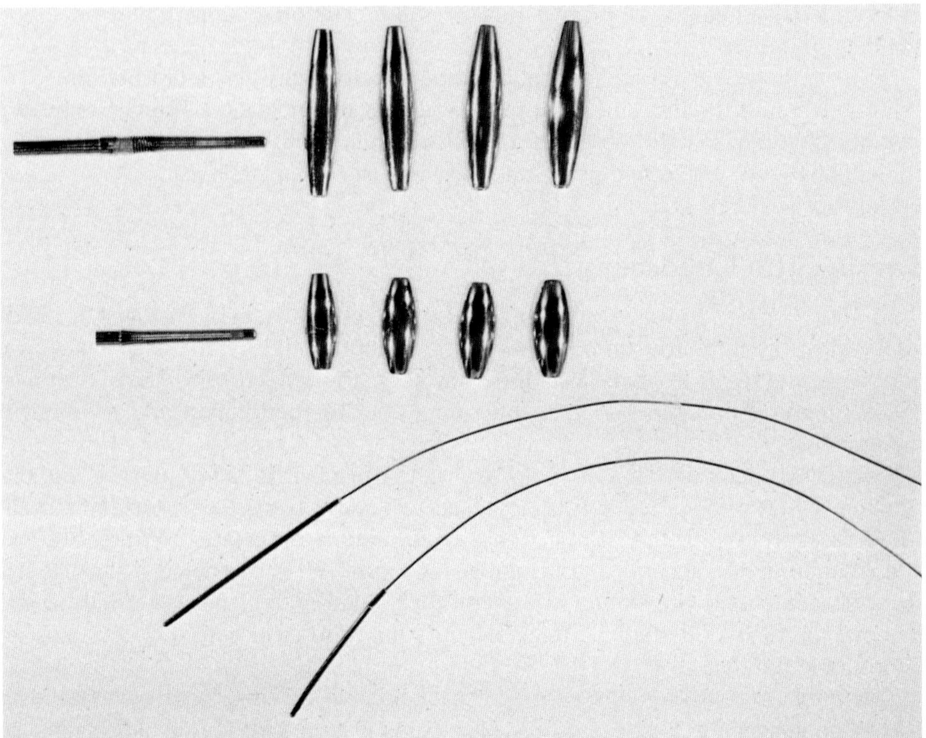

Figure 6-11. *Comparison between adult and miniaturized devices for esophageal dilatation (Eder-Puestow system).*

and caution must be used in inserting the fiberscope in underweight infants or respiratory-distressed children.

The main contraindication to fiberendoscopy in childhood is the overenthusiastic, inexperienced endoscopist.

In the case of massive hemorrhage, endoscopic examination must not interfere with the necessary and prompt emergency supportive measures.[21]

In some patients with severe psychological disturbances, the benefit of a diagnostic examination might be minimal compared to a major psychological trauma; this must therefore be considered as a contraindication.

Table 6-3
Esophageal Dilatations

Indications	No. Children	No. Dilatations
Congenital atresia	5	31
Peptic stenosis	3	14
Caustic stenosis	3	90
Radiation stricture	1	2
Extrinsic compression	1	2

Endoscopic Findings

Normal esophagus. The esophageal mucosa has a pale pink coloration and appears smooth, showing a fine vascular pattern. The normal cardia is usually closed but can be slightly opened either by normal peristaltic movements or by insufflation of air at a close distance. At the level of the cardial ring, the gastric mucosa with its more reddish coloration has an irregular delimitation from the esophageal mucosa.[23]

Peptic esophagitis. This pattern may lead to confusion in cases of mild esophagitis where the esophageal mucosa appears reddened and sometimes edematous with loss of the normal vascular pattern. Guided biopsies of the suspected zones are useful in distinguishing hyperemic esophagus from normal gastric mucosa. At a more advanced stage of esophagitis, the mucosa becomes friable and bleeds easily on touching and there are patches of exudate and ulcerations limited to the distal 3–4 cm of the esophagus (see Figure 19, p. v). More severe changes consist of larger ulcerated areas with heavy exudative lesions, sometimes separated by zones of pseudopolypoid mucosa. Most often these severe lesions are distributed along the distal third, but they can extend to the whole esophagus. These changes usually occur in children with a large hiatal hernia, incompetent lower esophageal sphincter, and abnormally shortened esophagus. The cardial ring is normally closed, but in cases of sliding hernia it appears constantly open, and respiratory movements are accompanied by an up-and-down sliding of the gastric folds above the diaphragmatic ring. When the tip of the fiberscope is inserted into the stomach, a U-turn maneuver of the bending tip by accentuating the "up" and "left" position places the optical tip in front of the gastric part of the cardia; this retrovision permits demonstration of the shaft of the instrument passing loosely through the hiatal zone and the pouch of gastric mucosa herniating above the diaphragmatic hiatus[23] (see Figure 20, p. v). In advanced cases, peptic stenosis is the final result. It can extend from the cardial zone upward along several cm or may spare the cardia itself and extend above this region. As in other types of strictures, dilatation under endoscopic control is indicated (see following text).

Caustic esophagitis. In milder cases, such as those occurring with ingestion of bleach, the mucosa is hyperemic with little or no edema or ulceration. On the other hand, in more severe cases, such as following ingestion of lye or ammonia, the mucosa is edematous at an early stage; but very soon after, the desquamating mucosa is replaced by a fibrinous material and ulcerations. The period extending from day 2 to day 8 is particularly delicate, and endoscopy should be performed under general anesthesia and with extreme caution. Cicatrization leads to strictures, generally asymmetrical, within 3–8 weeks, and one should be ready to perform dilatations as soon as possible.[15]

Scars. Mallory-Weiss syndrome, by laceration of the cardia after forceful vomiting, is rarer in children than in adults. The longitudinal fissure, usually at the level of the posterior wall of the cardia, can be better explored from the gastric side of the cardia by the retrovision technique. Other traumatic lacerations of the esophagus can occur in the upper third following ingestion of foreign bodies such as chicken bones or needles.

Varices. In cases of portal hypertension one can find either obvious varices lying in the long axis of the esophagus as tortuous bluish folds covered with otherwise normal mucosa or, in minor cases, more discrete hyperemia. It is important to investigate the stomach also, and in some cases varices can even be found in the duodenum.

Normal stomach. Gastric folds vary in size, and the endoscopic assessment depends greatly upon the degree of gastric distension. In infants they disappear almost completely after insufflation and the vascular pattern is easily seen, the coloration being paler than in older children and in adults.

Acute gastritis. The lesions consist of a generalized reddening of the mucosa; in some cases congestion of the mucosa alternates with multiple small erosions, giving a "salt-and-pepper" appearance. When the endoscopic findings are described, such terms as *edema, hyperemia, erosion,* and *ulceration* should be used instead of *gastritis,* which is proper only for those lesions in which a histologic confirmation can be obtained.

Chronic gastritis. In a few cases of children complaining of abdominal pain, small round polypoid lesions can be seen infiltrating the submucosa. These lesions are prominent at the level of the antrum, in our experience, but others have observed them invading the whole gastric cavity. The mucosa is either normal or hyperemic with small smooth umbilicated lesions. This condition can be observed together with gastric or duodenal ulcers but is also seen in the absence of other lesions (see Table 6-4). The significance of this so-called *état mamelonné* or pseudopolypoid gastritis resembling adult verrucous gastritis is poorly understood. Biopsies show mild to severe inflammatory changes, sometimes with an eosinophilic infiltration and hyposideremic anemia. Basal acid output is usually normal but may be either normal or decreased after pentagastrin stimulation. Complement deposits have been observed in rare cases[16] (Table 6-4).

Erosions and ulcers. These are the commonest localized lesions. Small, shallow lesions with no sign of scarring are called erosions, whereas more extensive and deep lesions are called ulcers (see Figures 21 and 22, p. vi). The prepyloric region and the duodenal bulb are the most frequent sites for solitary ulcers; however,

Table 6-4
Chronic Gastritis

Solitary Lesion	Associated Lesions
15 females/6 males	1 female/4 males: duodenal ulcers, duodenitis, Crohn's disease, cirrhosis

Total number 26, age 6 to 15 years, mean age 11.4 years
Family history of peptic ulcer in 6 cases

multiple ulcers are not rare, even in infancy. The lesion appears less profound in infants than in teenagers. Large extended ulcers, ringing the pylorus, may also be seen and may lead to scarring and stenosis. Radiation of mucosal folds toward the center of an ulcer is rarely observed in childhood. Edema and acute congestion surrounding the ulcerated duodenal mucosa are very helpful in indicating the central area, which might otherwise be difficult to localize in the duodenal bulb (Table 6-5).

Duodenitis. Small areas of mucosal congestion with spotty white exudate (salt-and-pepper mucosa) indicate duodenitis and can be the source of massive bleeding. The size of ulcerations, or even erosions, does not at all correlate with the importance of the bleeding (see Figures 23 and 24, p. vi).

Hypertrophic pyloric stenosis. In a few cases with secondary esophagitis and bleeding due to HPS, the pylorus appears narrowed with herniation of the pyloric mucosa extruding into the gastric cavity. In cases of incomplete stenosis of the pylorus, exaggeration and asymmetry of the folds is observed in the vicinity of the lesion.

Rare lesions. These are either fortuitous discoveries during a routine diagnostic examination or secondary to a previous radiologic study for confirmation or biopsy purposes. In our series, rare lesions include lymphoma of the duodenum with biliary fistula, congenital duodenal web, esophageal diverticulum, generalized polyposis of the stomach and duodenum, gastric angiomata, Peutz-Jeghers polyposis, Crohn's granulomata, and lymphoid hyperplasia of the duodenum.

ERCP is essentially a radiographic technique of opacification of the bile and/or pancreatic ducts that requires a skillful endoscopist for cannulation of the papilla and a trained radiologist for interpretation of the opacified anatomic structures. It remains a rare finding in childhood:[18,19] during one period only 26 children aged 9 months to 16 years were examined in collaboration with our adult endoscopy department (Prof. M. Cremer), whereas more than 5000 adults underwent an ERCP. Indications include chronic pancreatitis, congenital choledochal cyst, congenital abnormalities of the bile and pancreatic ducts, gallstones and choledochal stones, and invading lymphoma (see Chapter 7).

Table 6-5
Ulcers

Neonates and Infants, total number 7, age birth to 2 months			
Age less than 2 days	4	Age 15 days to 2 months	3
Esophagitis and gastric ulcers	4	Duodenal ulcers	2
		HPS	2
Infants and Children, total number 38, age 4 months to 15 years			
Gastric ulcers	19	Duodenal ulcers	19
Mean age 4.8 years		Mean age 11 years	
14 males/5 females		12 males/7 females	
Bleeding	14	Pain	11

References

1. Kawai K, Murakami K, Misak F: Endoscopical observations on gastric ulcers in teenagers. Endoscopy 2:206–208, 1970
2. Ottenjann R: Gastroscopic extraction of a foreign body. Endoscopy 3:193–194, 1970
3. Cremer M, Peeters JP, Emonts P, et al: Fiberendoscopy of the gastrointestinal tract in children: experience with newly designed fiberscopes. Endoscopy 6:186–189, 1974
4. Rodesch P, Cadranel S, Peeters JP, et al: Digestive endoscopy with fiberoptics in children, in Proceedings of the European Society of Paediatric Gastroenterology, Helsinki, August 1973. Abstracted, Acta Paediatr Scand 63:664, 1974
5. Gleason PD, Tedesco FJ, Keating WA: Fiberoptic gastrointestinal endoscopy in infants and children. J Pediatr 85:810–813, 1974
6. Gans SL, Ament ME, Christie DL: Pediatric endoscopy with flexible fiberscopes. J Pediatr Surg 10:375–380, 1975
7. Tedesco FJ, Goldstein PD, Gleason WA: Upper gastrointestinal endoscopy in pediatric patients. Gastroenterology 70:492–494, 1976
8. Cadranel S, Rodesch P, Peeters JP, et al: Fiberendoscopy of the gastrointestinal tract in children and infants: a series of 100 examinations. Am J Dis Child 131:41–45, 1977
9. Ament ME, Christie DL: Upper gastrointestinal fiberoptic endoscopy in pediatric patients. Gastroenterology 72:1244–1248, 1977
10. Burdelski M, Huchzermeyer H: Gastrointestinale Endoscopie im Kindesalter. Berlin, Springer-Verlag, 1980
11. Cremer N, Cadranel S, Rodesch P, et al: Paediatric gastrointestinal fiberendoscopy, in Current Concepts in Paediatric Radiology. Berlin/Heidelberg, Springer-Verlag, 1977
12. Mougenot JF, Polonowski C: Apport de la fibroscopie à la gastroentérologie pédiatrique. Le Pédiatre 50:7, 1975
13. Axon TR, Cotton PB, Philips I, et al: Disinfection of gastrointestinal fiberscopes. Lancet 1:656–658, 1974
14. Cadranel S, Rodesch P, Peeters JP, et al: Operative endoscopy in children. Acta Paediatr Belg 30:249, 1977
15. Cadranel S, Rodesch P, Peeters JP, et al: Fiberendoscopic monitorized dialtations of esophageal strictures in children. Endoscopy 9:127–130, 1977
16. Cadranel S, Rodesch P: Interest of endoscopic techniques in a paediatric gastroenterologic unit. Med Surg Ped 2:113–122, 1980
17. Forget PP, Meradji M: Contribution of fiberoptic endoscopy to diagnosis and management of children with gastroesophagel reflux. Arch Dis Child 51:60–66, 1976
18. Burdelski M, Huchzermeyer H: Diagnostic value of ERCP in children and adolescents, in Proceedings of the European Society for Paediatric Gastroenterology and Nutrition. Abstracted, Acta Paediatr Belg 32:153, 1979
19. Manegold BC, Joppich I: Laparoscopy and ERCP in children. Z Kinderchir (suppl) 27:125, 1979
20. Spencer R: Gastrointestinal hemorrhage in infancy and childhood. Surgery 55:718–734, 1964
21. Cadranel S, Rodesch P, Cremer N: Early fiberendoscopy in upper gastrointestinal tract bleeding in children. Acta Paediatr Belg 31:107, 1978
22. Christie DL, Ament ME: Removal of foreign bodies from esophagus and stomach with flexible fiberoptic panendoscopes. Pediatrics 57:931–934, 1976
23. Cotton PB, Williams CB: Practical Gastrointestinal Endoscopy. Oxford, Blackwell, 1980

Endoscopic Retrograde Cholangiopancreatography (ERCP)

CHAPTER 7

Hans Huchzermeyer

A wide spectrum of techniques yielding pictorial information, but varying in their potential, is available for the diagnosis of biliopancreatic diseases. The choice of an appropriate method should thus be dependent not only on its intrinsic value but also on the experience of the investigator and on the available technical setup. Moreover, it is preferable, particularly in children, to employ noninvasive techniques, at the same time avoiding radiation load or at least keeping it at a minimum. Of the direct methods, endoscopic retrograde cholangiopancreatography (ERCP) and also percutaneous transhepatic cholangiography (PTC) have become routine methods for diagnosis for adults. In pediatrics, however, experience with these techniques is as yet quite limited.[1–7,14] To date, intraoperative cholangiography and pancreatography have been given preference. Our own experience is based on the results of investigation in 36 children and juveniles in the age groups of 6 weeks to 14 years (23) and 15 to 18 years (13).

Instrumentation

Because of the anatomic conditions, special side-viewing instruments are best suited for inspection of the postbulbous duodenum and intubation of the papilla of Vater. The short point of this instrument is movable at two levels; the side-viewing optics

Table 7-1
Technical Data of Current ERCP Side-Viewing Instruments

	Olympus JF-B 2	Fujinon/C DUO-X	ACMI TX-6
Total length (mm)	1520	1500	1510
Working length (mm)	1370	1340	1200
Cross-section of the flexible part (mm)	10.0	11	10.0
Fixed point part			
Length (mm)	17.0	17	17.0
Diameter (mm)	10.0	17	10.0
Angle of view field	65°		65°
Depth of focus (mm)	5–60	2–80	5–80
Bending angle of the clamp	30°–85°	up to 85°	up to 90°
Bending angle of the point			
Upward	120°	120°	140°
Downward	120°	120°	140°
To the right	90°	90°	110°
To the left	90°	90°	110°

can be cleaned by an automatic washing and suction arrangement. Various models of adult duodenoscopes are available (Table 7-1); a special instrument for the pediatric age group has not been available as yet.

Technique

Up to the age of 10–12 years, ERCP should be carried out under intubation anesthesia; older boys and girls can be premedicated with sedatives or analgesics and atropine. The indication for sedation or anesthesia should not, however, be determined according to a rigid scheme. The behavior and wishes of the children should be taken into account. The investigation is done on an inpatient basis since a 3-day observation period is necessary afterwards.

The duodenoscope is advanced to the antrum with the patient on his left side or in the prone position. After engaging the pylorus, the instrument is flexed ventrally and introduced into the bulb of the duodenum. After clockwise rotation and further advancement, one finally arrives in the descending duodenum. Here, as a rule, the papilla is found in the proximal half of the small curvature; it is often marked by a longitudinal mucous fold that runs distally toward it. The papilla itself is flat or papillous, with a centrally situated ostium. However, the position and form of the papilla and the position of the ostium can vary greatly. In 20–50 percent of patients a minor papilla is observed above the major papilla, but this can seldom be probed. As in the stomach, little air is insufflated into the duodenum to avoid stimulating peristaltic action. Sedation of the duodenum is possible by intravenous injection of glucagon or hyoscine-*N*-butyl bromide. After introduction of the catheter (in the case of a small ostium, the catheter can often only be placed onto it), the contrast medium is instilled, the examiner observing the screen continuously, whereupon probing from either the horizontal or from the more distal direction results in filling predominantly the pancreatic duct or the bile duct, respectively. Filling, taut-filling, and emptying phases are recorded in general survey and specifically aimed exposures. Late pictures (up to 30 minutes and more) can be particularly valuable, for example, in revealing concrements or determining emptying time.

The technique of investigation in children and juveniles does not differ from that in adults. In neonates, however, the investigation is more complicated because of the large diameter of the usual side-viewing instruments. On the one hand, the papilla is placed relatively high in the duodenum; on the other, the distance from the instrument to the papilla is very short, thus hindering directing of the catheter. Introduction into the ostium consequently succeeds more often from a more horizontal than a distal direction, so that the pancreatic duct is displayed more than the bile duct. Simplication of the technique and therefore a better success rate can be expected in the future, after the development of thinner duodenoscopes.

Indications

An indication for ERCP is generally present if the diagnosis of a bile duct–gallbladder disease or pancreatic disease has not been definitely confirmed by the history, physical examination, and clinical-chemical studies, sonography, indirect cholangiography, and possibly also hepatobiliary sequence scintigraphy and computer tomography (Table 7-2).

In childhood, cholestasis syndrome presents a particular indication for ERCP. In infants and children, congenital anomalies are the main etiology; in juveniles, as in young adults, cholelithiasis and benign bile duct obstructions not caused by stones, but of inflammatory origin, are the most frequent reasons. Secondary stenosis in inflammatory disease of the pancreas also belongs to this group. In endemic regions such as South Africa, cholestasis due to parasite (Ascaris) infestation of the bile ducts can occasionally play a role.[8]

The fact that ERCP should not be considered at the outset but rather at the conclusion of diagnostic studies is particularly valid for its application in pancreatic disorders. It is true that, in individual cases, the cause of recurring acute pancreatitis can occasionally be found, or evidence of the respective duct deformities can confirm the suspected diagnosis of chronic pancreatitis. In such cases, however, ERCP is indicated only if surgical consequences are to be expected from the result. This is particularly true since, with sonography, a method is available to demonstrate acute pancreatitis and its complications, such as cysts, abscess, and necrosis formation, and in most cases is also able to identify chronic pancreatitis.

Table 7-2
Indications for Performing ERCP in Children

Cholestasis and obstructive jaundice (anatomic anomalies of the biliary system, cholelithiasis, inflammation and scar obstructions of the bile duct)
Acute recurrent pancreatitis; chronic pancreatitis
Suspicion of hemobilia or rupture of the pancreas (blunt abdominal trauma)
Pancreatic anomalies (annular pancreas)

In rare instances, the occurrence of upper intestinal bleeding following blunt abdominal trauma with suspicion of hemobilia or rupture of the pancreas can be an indication for ERCP. Similarly, suspicion of an anomaly of the pancreas can present a further rare indication. Here, only annular pancreas has clinical relevance, as it is the only symptomatic anomaly.

ERCP should be carried out in children only by an investigator experienced with endoscopy in adults, in cooperation with an experienced pancreas and bile duct surgeon.

Contraindications

Since in individual cases one cannot definitely predict which duct system will be filled, it follows that acute pancreatitis, pseudocysts of the pancreas, and acute cholangitis with stenotic processes are the most important contraindications (Table 7-3).

Following an attack of acute pancreatitis or an acute phase of chronic pancreatitis, ERCP should (with sonographic monitoring) be carried out no sooner than 4 weeks for the clarification of drainage conditions. If one suspects such a drainage obstruction in one of the two duct systems, a broad spectrum antibiotic should be given prophylactically and the investigation carried out with preparation for surgery so that if an obstruction is demonstrated it can be removed rapidly by an operation.

Because of problems in complete sterilization of endoscopes, one should dispense with ERCP in patients with an HBs-antigenemia because of possible infection of other patients.

Complications

With proper technique and observation of the above contraindications, the complication rate in the pediatric age group should be just as low as in adults. With the small number of children investigated to date, there are no precise data for this.

Success Rate

Because of a numerically limited experience, there are also no statements to date regarding the success rate of ERCP in the pediatric age group. In children and juveniles (but not necessarily in infants), the success rate should be comparable with

Table 7-3
Contraindications for Performing ERCP in Children

Contraindications for Performing ERCP in Children
Acute pancreatitis; active phase of a chronic pancreatitis
Pancreas pseudocyst
Acute cholangitis
Acute viral hepatitis, HBs-antigenemia
Contraindications for proximal intestinoscopy

that in adults. Filling of one or both duct systems, according to our own experience (3500 ERCPs since 1971), succeeded in 84 percent of cases (results in the literature vary between 62 percent and 97 percent).

The Normal Cholangiogram and Pancreatogram

Recognition of the normal cholangiogram and pancreatogram is the prerequisite for efficient diagnosis and differentiation of various diseases (Figures 7-1, 7-2). Age-dependent variations of the diameters of the two duct systems must, however, be emphasized. With increasing age, and thus with increasing organ size, there is a continuous increase in caliber of each section of the bile duct system. The widest diameter is found in the region of the supraduodenal part of the common duct, while the other sections have a smaller diameter. The nature of the ducts is such that wide individual variations in caliber occur. The data presented in Table 7-4, however, give the maximal values for juveniles.

Length and diameter of the pancreatic duct largely correlate with the size of the pancreas and also increase continuously with advancing age of the child (with individual variations). From our own investigations, we summarize data as maximal values for juveniles in Table 7-5. The pancreatic duct narrows continuously from head to tail. First-order branches can reach a length of 1–2 cm and a caliber of 0.1–0.3 mm. The drainage time of the contrast medium from the bile duct system should be, at the most, 20 to 30 minutes, and from the pancreatic duct system, 3 to 5 minutes. Longer drainage times should be viewed as abnormal.

Congenital Malformations and Diseases of the Bile Ducts

Numerous varieties of congenital anomalies of the bile ducts can be observed. However, only bile duct atresia and congenital dilation of the bile ducts are of clinical significance. Rapid diagnosis of congenital bile duct atresia is still a problem. So far as ERCP is concerned, the development of narrower pediatric endoscopes would be necessary for satisfactory use in this diagnosis.

Congenital dilatation of the bile ducts can occur both in the small intrahepatic and in the large intra- and extrahepatic bile ducts. ERCP plays no role in the diagnosis of the closely related deformities of the small bile ducts and is involved only in dilatation of the large intrahepatic and extrahepatic bile ducts.[3,9–13]

Three forms of cystic choledochal dilatation are differentiated according to site and form:

1. Choledochal cyst
2. Choledochal diverticulum
3. Choledochocele

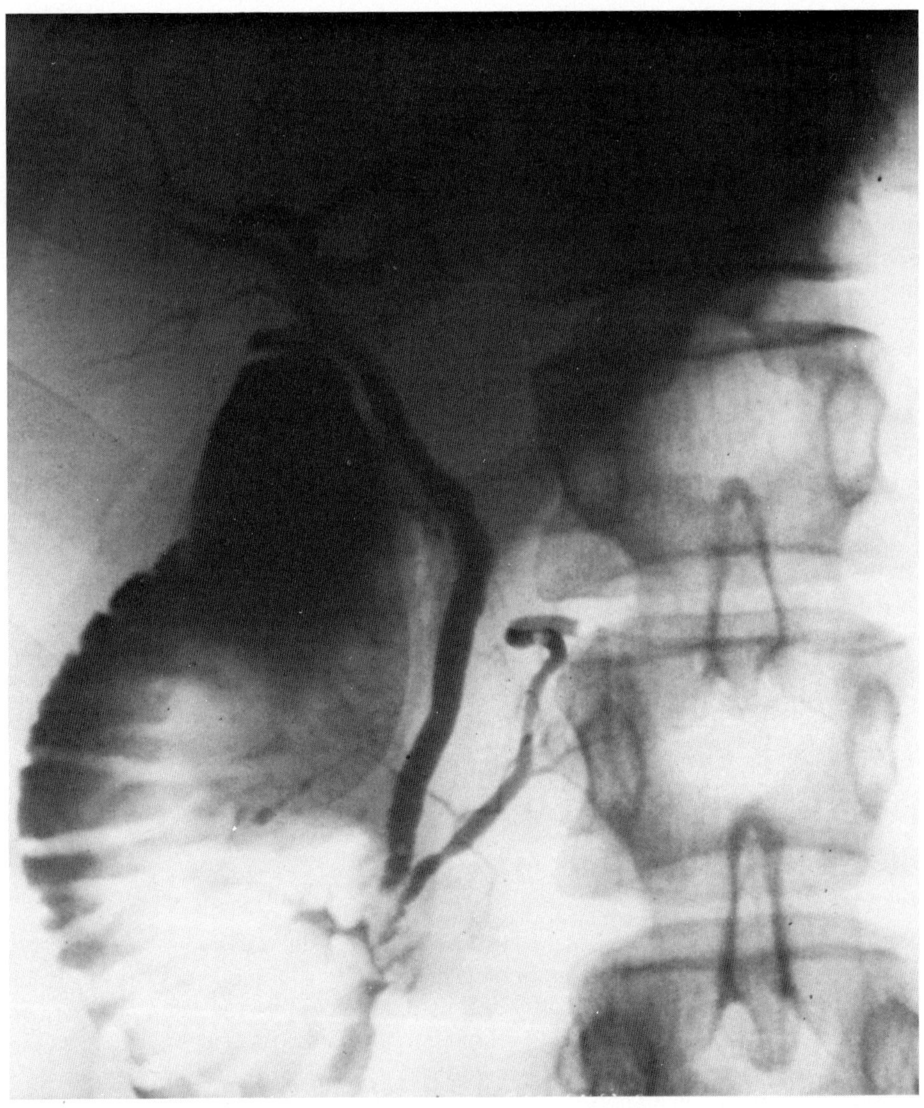

Figure 7-1. *Normal cholangiopancreatogram. Narrow common duct and hepatic ducts, delicate branching of the intrahepatic bile ducts. Filling of the gall bladder via the cystic duct. Delicate duct of Santorini.*

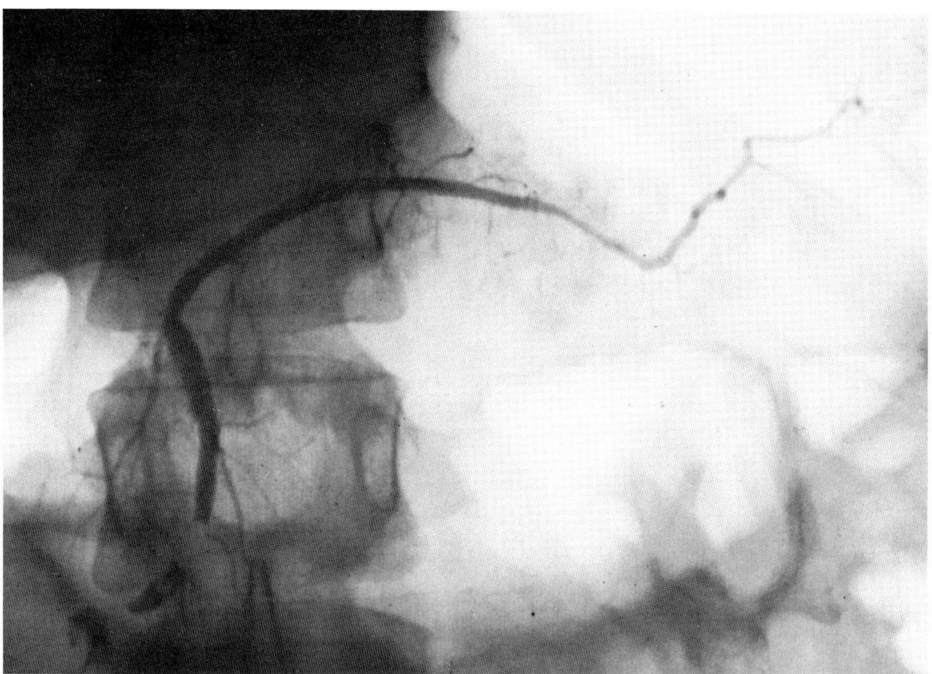

Figure 7-2. *Normal pancreatic duct system (Wirsung's duct, Santorini's duct, and numerous pancreatic branches).*

Table 7-4
Diameter of the Bile Duct System (mm) in the Endoscopic Retrograde Cholangiogram of 21 Normal Persons 15–25 Years Old (M ± SEM)

Ductus choledochus	
Pars pancreatica	3.8 ± 0.4 mm
Pars supraduodenalis	4.4 ± 0.5 mm
Ductus hepaticus	
Communis	3.5 ± 0.6 mm
Sinister/dexter	2.9 ± 0.4 mm
Interlobular bile ducts	2.0 ± 0.5 mm

Table 7-5
Lengths and Diameters of the Pancreatic Duct in Endoscopic Retrograde Pancreatograms in 11 Normal Persons 16–24 Years Old (M ± SEM)

Pancreatic Duct	Diameter (mm)	Length (cm)
Head	3.3 ± 0.5	
Body	1.7 ± 0.3	15.1 ± 0.3
Tail	1.5 ± 0.3	

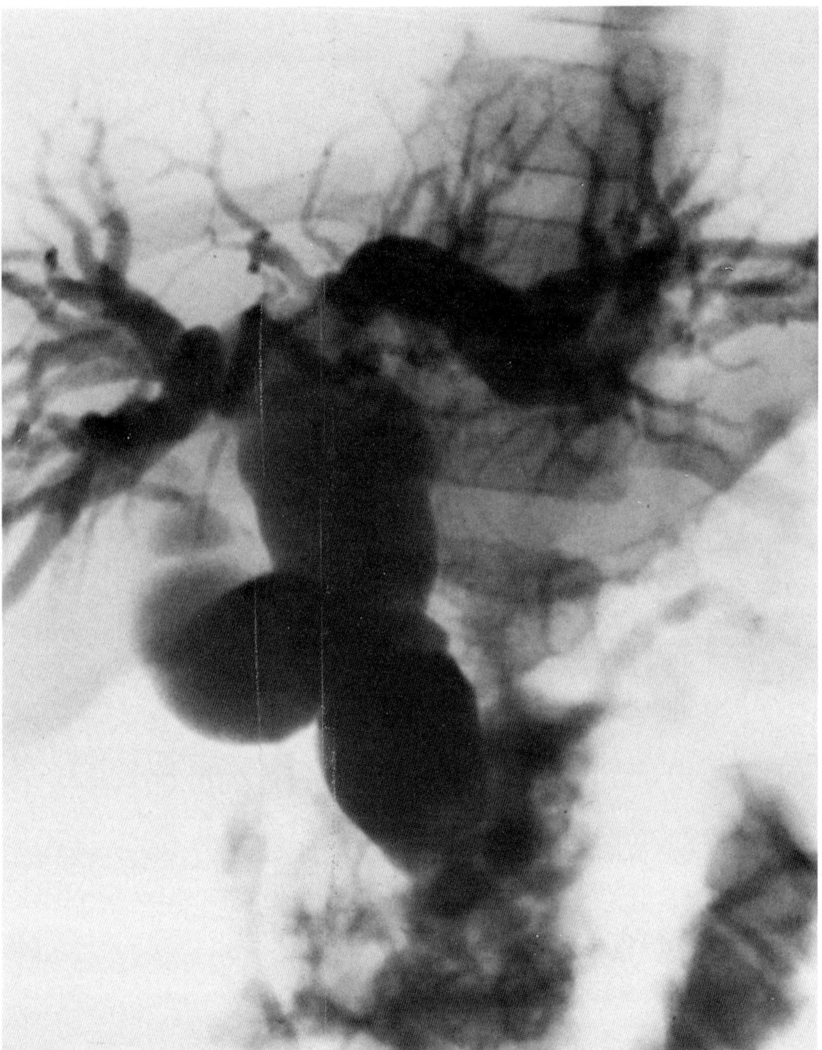

Figure 7-3. *A 4-year-old girl with a choledochal cyst. Retrograde cholangiogram of the common duct, which is enlarged up to 22 mm. Dilatation of the right and left hepatic ducts and a laterally placed gallbladder. Common junction with the slightly enlarged pancreatic duct. As a complication of ERCP, appearance of cholangitis and pancreatitis with septic temperatures. Operative excision of the cysts and the gallbladder with application of a hepatojejunostomy Roux-Y.*

With the aid of sonography the size, form, and site, as well as the liquid content of the cyst, can be seen with good reliability from a lumen width of about 1 cm.[9] However, in order to be able to recognize the extent of the dilatation with certainty, and to assess exactly the distal segment of the common duct and its relationship to the pancreatic duct, ERCP is indicated.

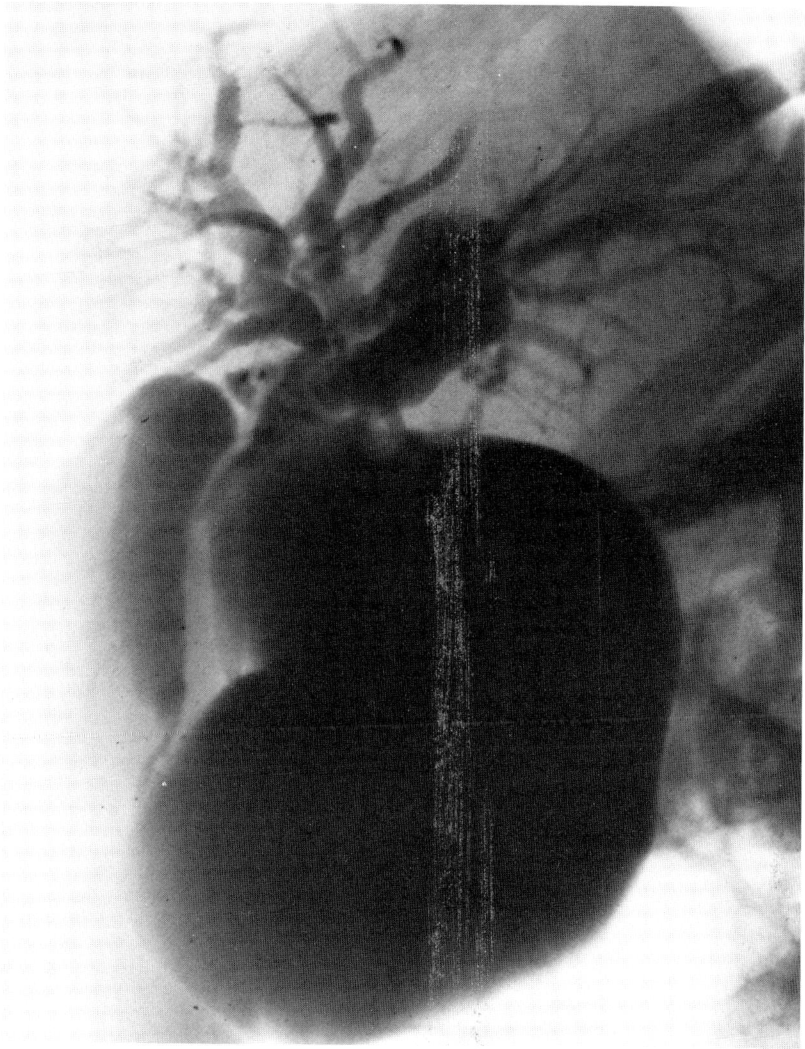

Figure 7-4. *A 12-year-old boy with a choledochal cyst. Retrograde cholangiogram of the massively enlarged common duct, which leads into intrahepatic bile ducts of virtually normal caliber. Laterally with respect to the cyst is the enlarged gallbladder. Absence of release of contrast medium into the duodenum. Selective visualization of an inconspicuous pancreatic duct.*

Since this procedure allows the instillation of sufficient contrast medium, the various types of cyst can be well depicted (Figures 7-3, 7-4). It is important that abnormal connections of the pancreaticobiliary duct system be excluded. The pancreatic duct can flow into the bile duct or, clinically more serious, the bile duct can flow into the pancreatic duct. Only with a precise knowledge of the topographic relationships of the two duct systems can the surgical tactics be determined in advance, and only in this way can the otherwise necessary intraoperative cholangiography be avoided. Here, PTC is inferior to ERCP, since it contrasts only the bile duct system, and should be applied only in the event of failure of ERCP.

Acquired Disorders of the Bile Duct

Not only congenital disorders of the bile duct but also acquired disorders are among the uncommon diseases of childhood. These are observed more often in juveniles. As in early adulthood, extrahepatic cholestasis due to cholelithiasis or benign non-stone-originating bile duct obstructions are foremost.

The diagnosis of gallstones is made primarily by sonography and with excretion cholangiography. Thus, very few children need be subjected to further endoscopic (ERCP) or invasive (PTC) procedures.

Even rarer than cholelitheasis in childhood are the non-stone-originating obstructive bile duct alterations: scar strictures (after liver, bile duct, stomach, or pancreatic operations); pancreatic diseases (inflammation, carcinoma, pseudocyst); metastases; impressions of lymph nodes; abscesses; sclerotic cholangitis (Figure 7-5); papillary stenosis; parasites (*Ascaris, Fasciola hepatica, Echinococcus*, etc.); benign tumors of the bile duct (papilloma, adenoma, etc.); and carcinoma of the bile duct and gallbladder.

Finally, traumatic hemobilia and bilhemia are of increasing importance in children as a result of increasing numbers of traffic accidents. It is important to recognize the intrahepatic lesion without delay and to locate it exactly, as this determines the surgical procedure. The diagnosis is made by a combination of sonography, angiography, and ERCP (Figure 7-6). In additon, other causes of bleeding in the upper gastrointestinal tract (such as stress ulcer) can be excluded.

Congenital Malformation and Diseases of the Pancreas

Congenital anomalies of position, form, and size of the pancreas are rare and usually are asymptomatic. With annular pancreas, stenosis of the duodenum can be mild to severe. The diagnosis can be made by ERCP, since in the formation of the ring a pancreatic duct is always involved (Figure 7-7).

Acquired Disorders of the Pancreas

The various forms of pancreatitis are particularly worthy of mention here although considered rare in children. Because of the lack of valid methods of detection, they are only found by surgeons during exploratory laparotomy or by pathologists at autopsy. Special interest is devoted to acute and chronic pancreatitis, which can be caused and maintained by many diverse etiological factors. Blunt and penetrating

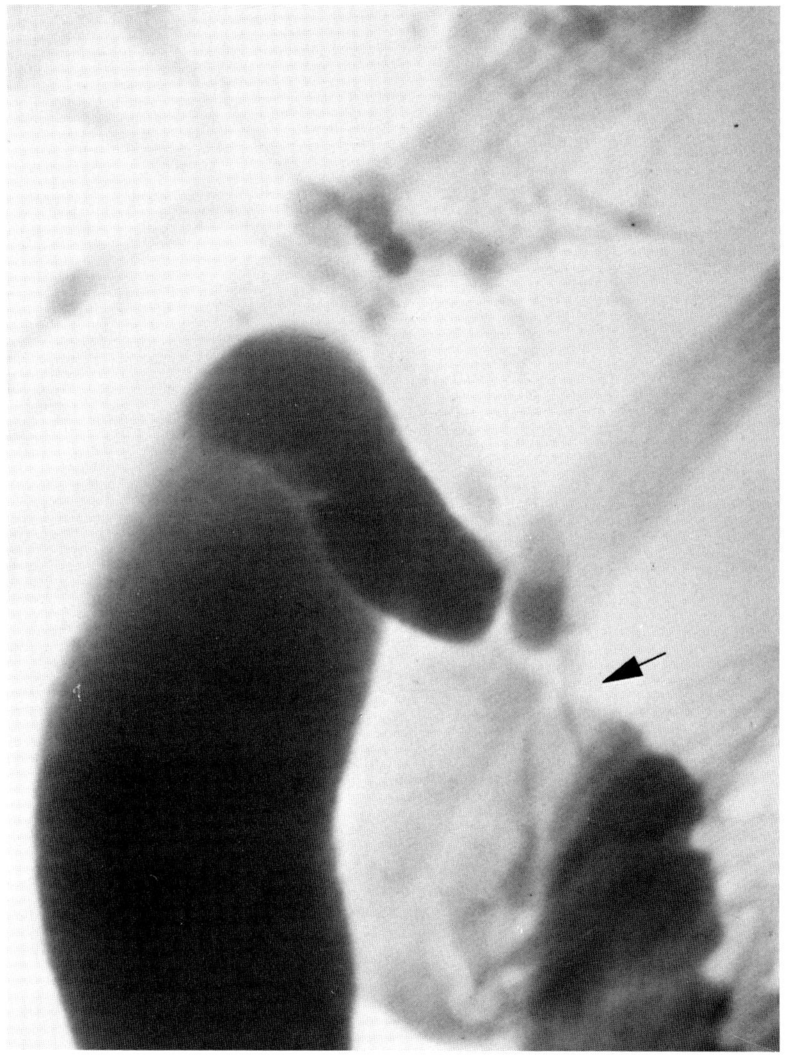

Figure 7-5. *A 16-year-old girl with sclerotic cholangitis in a retrograde cholangiogram. Irregularly defined stenosis of the common duct.*

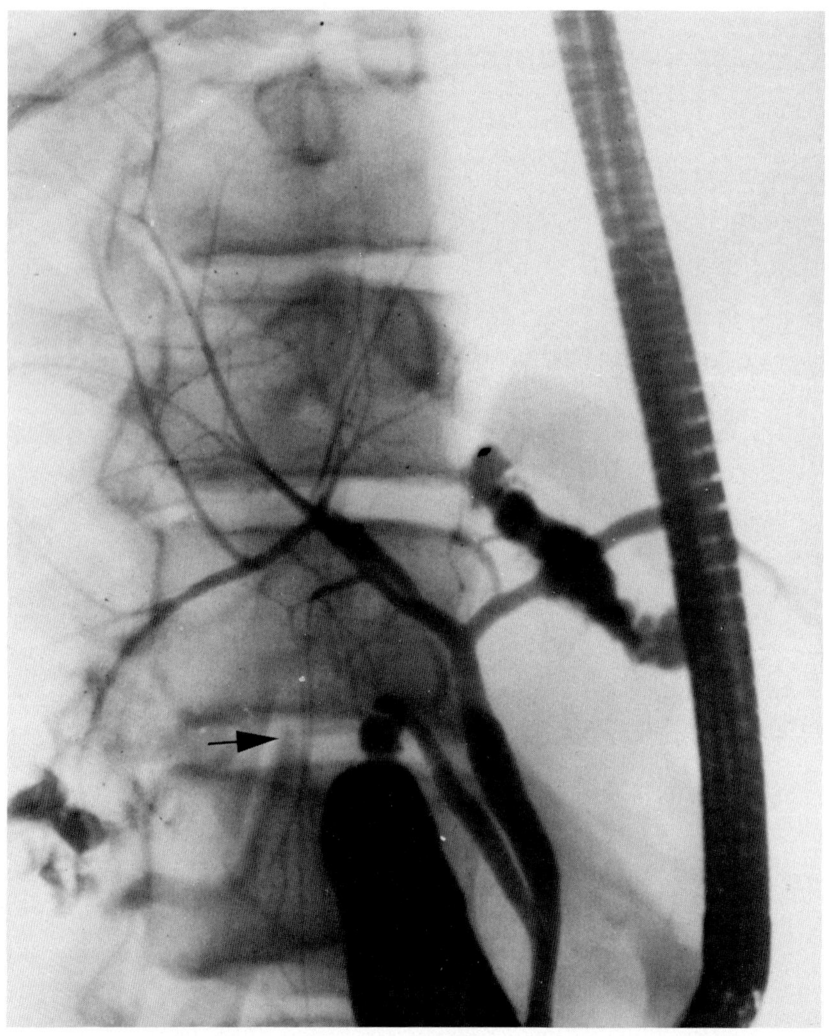

Figure 7-6. *ERC in traumatic bilhemia in a 15-year-old patient. Flow of contrast medium into the parenchyma of the left (from a side branch of the left hepatic duct) and right liver lobes with deflection of the bile ducts.*

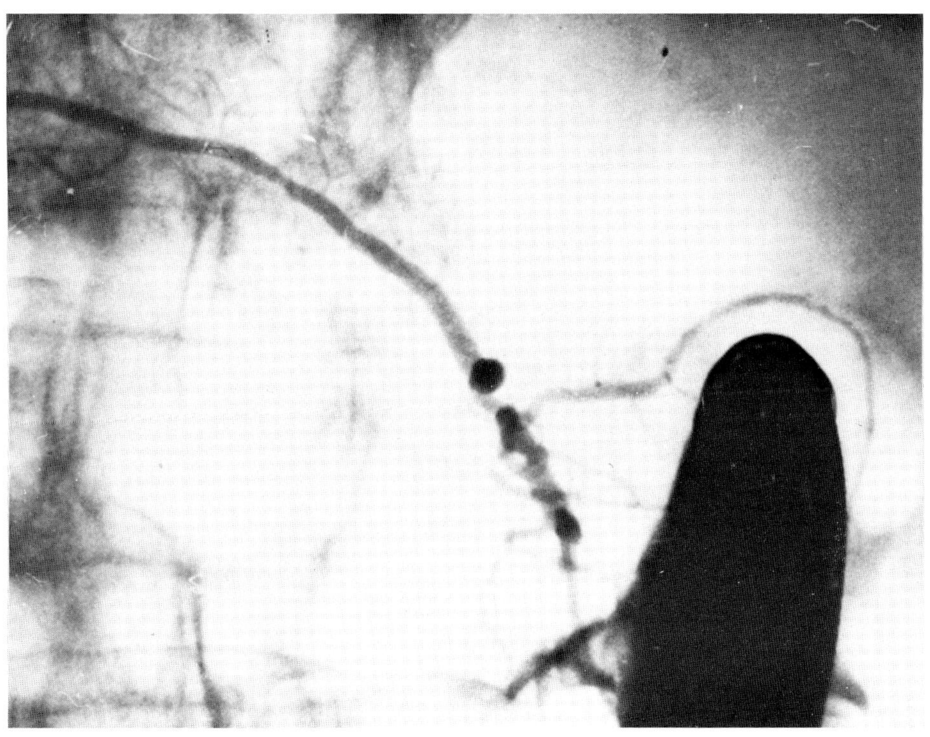

Figure 7-7. *Annular pancreas (ERP). The descending duodenum is partially surrounded by the ductus Santorini. (Courtesy of M. Classen, Frankfurt/Main, West Germany.)*

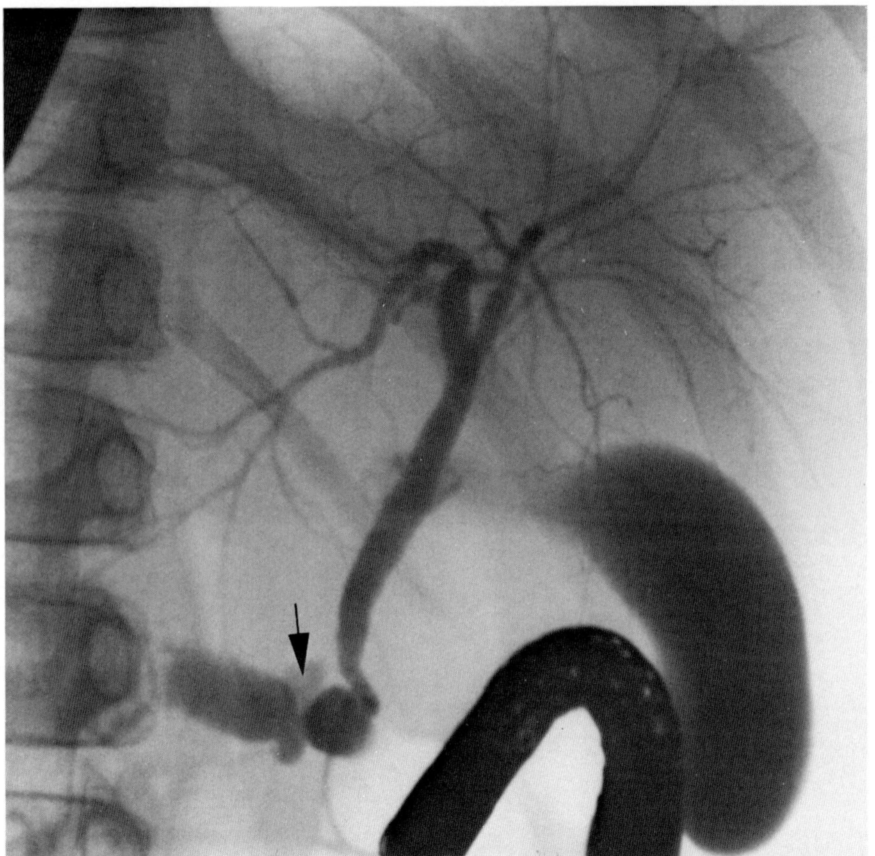

Figure 7-8. *Acute recurrent pancreatitis in a 9-year-old girl (ERCP). Transcribed stenosis of the pancreatic duct in the head region with prestenotic dilatation.*

abdominal trauma are rare causes of acute pancreatitis. Pressure of the pancreas against the vertebral column, however, can lead to rupture of the parenchyma, the duct system, or vessels. Further results are the formation of hematomas and the development of pseudocysts. For detection of these conditions, sonography, arteriography, and ERCP are useful. With ERCP, release of contrast medium from the duct system, possibly into small necrotic cavities, can be followed.[2,4–7,14]

Chronic pancreatitis is characterized pancreatographically by two typical findings: deformity of the duct system and pancreatic pseudocysts.

Since there is a danger of an infection of pseudocysts from ERCP and since these cysts can be detected by sonography, pseudocysts should appear only in exceptional cases as an unexpected finding in ERCP. Deformities of the duct system can appear in varying degrees of severity. If they are only of a mild nature, then there will be only slight segmental variations in caliber or stenosis of the main duct or isolated cystic enlargements of the side ducts. the pancreatic duct is not enlarged, and the release of the contrast medium is hardly or not at all delayed. In advanced changes, the whole duct system is affected. The main duct is noticeably enlarged and exhibits variations in caliber, cystic distention, and occasionally intraductally positioned

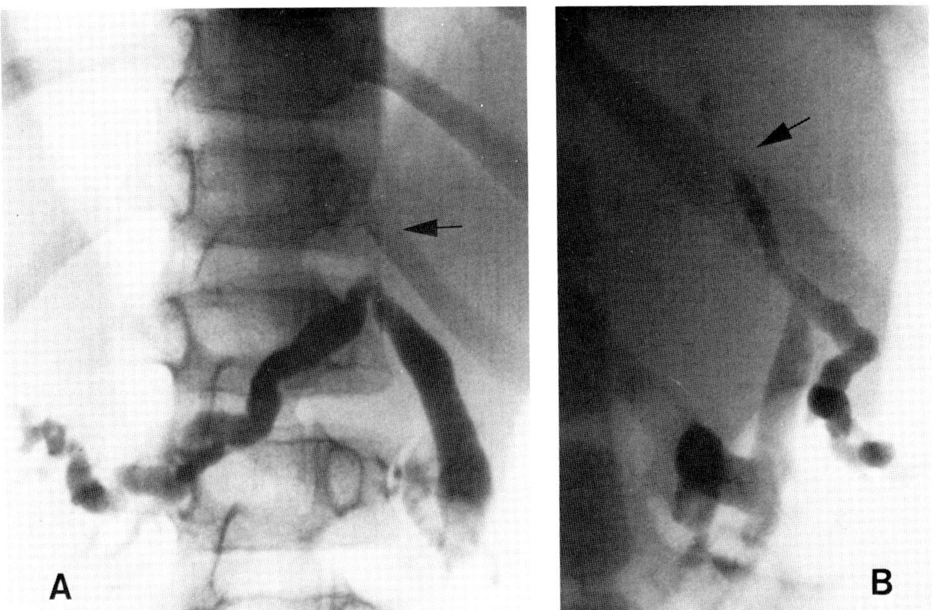

Figure 7-9. *(A) Acute recurrent pancreatitis in a 9-year-old boy (ERP). Deformity and dilatation of the main pancreatic duct. (B) Internal pancreatic fistula into the left pleural cavity with resultant pleural effusion.*

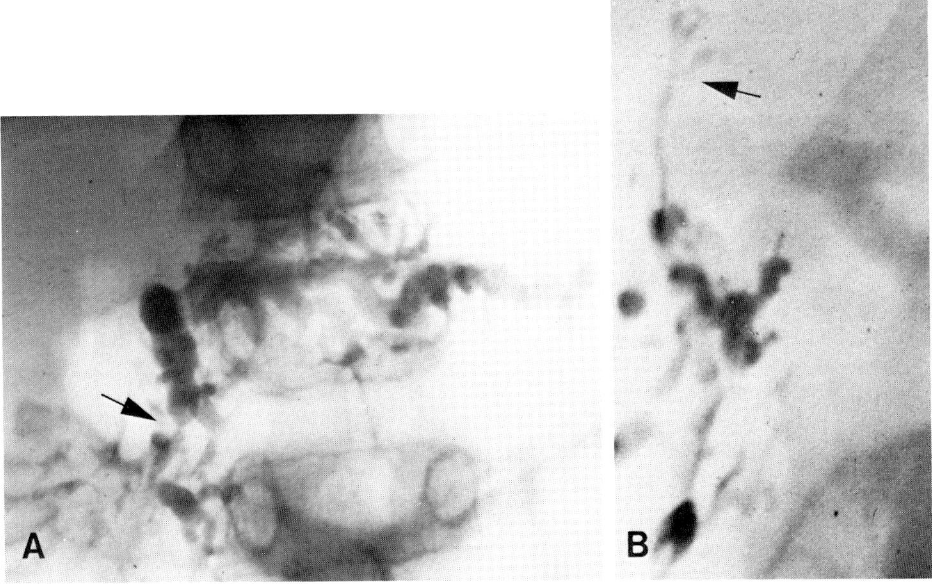

Figure 7-10. *Chronic recurrent pancreatitis in a 12-year-old boy (ERP). Stenosis of the pancreatic duct (A) and visualization of a small fistula entry in the head region (B), deformity and dilatation of the whole duct system, including the side branches. Clearly delayed release of the contrast medium (more than 2 hours).*

stones. In the side branches there are dilatations, cystic distention, and irregularities in caliber. Contrast-medium clearance can be extended by as much as 30 minutes or longer. High degrees of stenosis are relatively rare in the pancreatic duct with prestenotic enlargement of the duct system or even complete discontinuity (Figures 7-8, 7-9, 7-10). Pseudocysts of varying size, and located individually or multiply in the head, body, or tail regions, can be present both in discrete and in massive deformities of the ducts. A further complication of chronic pancreatitis can be stenosis of the common bile duct or the duodenal lumen.

Primary or metastic malignant tumors of the pancreas are extreme rarities in childhood. Pancreatographically, changes can be detectable according to the starting point and size of the tumor. Most commonly, the pancreatic duct exhibits a transcribed stenosis with or without prestenotic dilatation or a complete interruption of filling. On rare occasions one finds a gradual decrease in the pancreatic duct down to the tail region (tapering type). Unfortunately, these diagnostic characteristics are not early but are late symptoms and, furthermore, do not permit a definite differentiation from a chronic pancreatitis.

References

1. Burdelski M, Huchzermeyer H: Gastrointestinale Endoskopie im Kindesalter. Berlin, Springer-Verlag, 1981
2. Filston HC, McLeod ME, Bolman RM, et al: Improved management of pancreatic lesions in children aided by ERCP. J Pediatr Surg 15:121, 1980
3. Huchzermeyer H, Burdelski M, Gebel M: Diagnostische Bedeutung der endoskopischen retrograden Cholangio-Pankreatikografie und der perkutanen transhepatischen Feinnadelcholangiografie beim Cholestase-Syndrom im Kindesalter und Jugendalter. Leber Magen Darm 9:60, 1979
4. Riemann JF, Koch H: Endoscopy of the biliary tract and the pancreas in children. Endoscopy 10:166, 1978
5. Van der Spuy S: Endoscopic retrograde cholangiopancreatography (ERCP) in children. Endoscopy 10:173, 1978
6. Urakami Y, Seki H, Kishi S: Endoscopic retrograde cholangiopancreatography (ERCP) performed in children. Endoscopy 9:86, 1978
7. Waye JD: Endoscopic retrograde cholangiopancreatography in the infant. Am J Gastroenterol 65:461, 1976
8. Van der Spuy S: Biliary ascariasis—endoscopic aspects. S Afr Med J 53:1030, 1978
9. Gebel M, Huchzermeyer H: Die Sonografie in der Diagnostik des Cholestase-Syndroms im Kindesalter. Leber Magen Darm 9:65, 1979
10. Burcharth F, Huchzermeyer H, Burdelski M: Transhepatic and retrograde cholangiography in the diagnosis of biliary atresia (in preparation)
11. Caroli J: Diseases of the intrahepatic biliary tree. Clin Gastroenterol 2:147, 1973
12. Nelson R, Hamlyn AH, Lavelle I: Fine needle percutaneous transhepatic cholangiography in the investigation of cholestasis in infancy. J Pediatr Surg 12:727, 1977
13. Starzl TE: Liver replacement in children, in Berenberg SR: Liver Disease in Infancy and Childhood. Den Haag, Nijhoff, 1976, p 97
14. Vantini J, Piubello W, Ederle A, et al: Hereditary pancreatitis: morphological pictures (ERCP) in the youngest member of a family. Acta Hepato-Gastroenterol 26:253, 1979

Colonoscopy

CHAPTER 8

Christopher B. Williams
Samy Cadranel

Colonoscopy is technically a more difficult procedure than gastroscopy, although relatively easier in children than in adults, whose colons are more often bound down by postoperative or postinflammatory adhesions. Until now pediatric colonoscopes suitable for use in neonates or babies have not been available, which has undoubtedly inhibited many centers from buying instruments and using the technique. In the future there is every reason to think that colonoscopy will be as important a screening procedure in children as it is in adults. Limited examination with a thin fiberoptic instrument is kinder to the child than with a rigid proctosigmoidoscope; it looks farther and makes it very easy to take photographs or small biopsy specimens. Total colonoscopy is a more difficult procedure but more accurate than barium enema and will, therefore, be the procedure of choice in certain patients.

The relationship in pediatric practice between colonoscopy and barium enema could take some years to develop; at present relatively few centers perform either technique to a satisfactory standard. The barium enema by the air-contrast method is a refined and accurate technique compared to the crude single-contrast method employed in most x-ray departments for children. It is true that the necessary degree of air distention for a high-quality x-ray is uncomfortable, but so is colonoscopy, and the barium enema has the potential advantage over colonoscopy of providing a permanent record of the appearances of the whole colon. The photographs and even color video-tape record of colonoscopy give at best a partial view.

For certain purposes, such as showing the shape of the colon and demonstrating the extent of strictures or the presence of transmural fistulas and fissures, the barium enema is considerably superior to colonoscopy. Certainly the two examinations are to a large extent complementary, radiology for the overall view and endoscopy for fine detail and biopsy (including polypectomy). Which procedure is used will depend to some extent on local circumstances and, if both are equally available, on the information required from each particular examination. There are attractions in pediatric practice in obtaining at a single endoscopic procedure, without general anesthesia, proctosigmoidoscopy and examination of the proximal colon and terminal ileum with directed biopsies from representative areas. Pediatric radiologists will doubtless, as has happened in adult radiology, respond to the competitive stimulus of colonoscopy with improvements in their barium enema technique, thus reconfirming the importance of x-ray as the less invasive technique.

Instrumentation

Although adult colonoscopes are frequently and successfully used in pediatric practice,[1-10] insertion of a tip diameter of 15 mm is a hostile act not appreciated by small children. A pediatric colonoscope[2,3,9-11] should have a reduced diameter and a tip designed for easy insertion, the squamous epithelium of the anus being the only sensitive part of the bowel. Although the single-channel adult colonoscope is more flexible or "soft" than even the pediatric gastroscope, it is still relatively stiff and clumsy to the thin and elastic colon of young children; an adult instrument can reasonably be used on a well-developed 10-year-old, but neonates or small or frail children need the appropriately designed colonoscope.

The instrument manufacturers have now produced a number of different prototype pediatric instruments with varying characteristics, primarily smaller shaft diameter. An instrument that is thin but very stiff—such as all avaliable pediatric gastroscopes and some "pediatric" colonoscopes—is potentially traumatic in stretching the variable loops and bends of the colon. Pediatric gastroscopes may have too small a suction channel to aspirate residual bowel contents satisfactorily or may not have the forced water-washing syringe, which is essential to clean the instrument tip if bowel preparation is poor. The bending characteristics of pediatric gastroscopes are also far from ideal for colonoscopy. An acutely retroflexing tip tends to impact rather than pass easily around the splenic flexure, although a long "bending segment" makes angulation to the ileocecal valve of neonates impossible.

The ideal length for a pediatric instrument is debatable, but it is unlikely that more than 110–130 cm is necessary, since in a neonate the cecum is reached with about 50 cm of instrument and lies at only 30 cm when the colonoscope is straightened out. In small children, 80–90 cm may be needed to reach the cecum

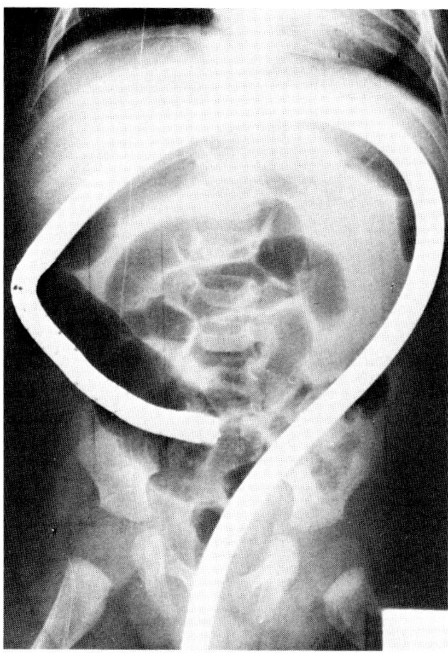

Figure 8-1. *Radiograph of total colonoscopy to the cecum in a 3-month-old child using a small-diameter pediatric colonoscope.*

and the colon shortens to 50 cm; the additional length of the instrument would allow for examination of older children and avoid the endoscopist getting a backache. In truth, it is unlikely that there will ever be a single ideal pediatric colonoscope suitable for all ages and all sizes of children. The best compromise may be to have a thin and floppy instrument suitable for babies and small children (Figure 8-1) that would be used for all limited examinations of older age groups, in whom total colonoscopy could either be performed using a suitable stiffening overtube under fluoroscopic control or by employing an adult or stiffer pediatric instrument.

Instrument Cleaning and Sterilization

As mentioned in chapter 7, physical care of small-diameter instruments[12] is of extreme importance, since they are even more fragile than larger instruments and their channels more liable to blockage. Either the endoscopist or a designated experienced nurse must know how to clean through the air, water, and suction channels and disassemble the suction port and its valve mechanism. Mechanical cleansing with cationic soaps, warm water, and alcohol, using suction, syringe, or pressure gun, channel brush, and toothbrush is the first step in antisepsis. Soaking in chlorhexidine in 30 percent alcohol and thorough drying can provide virtual sterility, but soaking in glutaraldehyde solution or ethylene oxide gas sterilization is necessary for greater security. The endoscope must also be recleaned *before* use to remove any bacterial growth that may have occurred during storage.

There have so far been no reports of infection transmitted via the colonoscope, but this is clearly a particular worry in pediatric practice.

Bowel Preparation

A clean colon, empty of solid stool and particulate food residue, is essential for successful colonoscopy. Whereas small babies, already on a fluid diet, are easy to prepare, large children need stronger measures. There is no ideal regime that is welcome to the patient and also effective, and every regime has its occasional failures. The preparation to be used is chosen both according to the age and physical condition of the child and to the extent of the intended examination. A single warm saline or hypertonic phosphate enema[5,10] should clean nearly all the colon of a neonate but only the distal colon of most older children. Those with diarrhea may need only a day on a clear fluid diet and one or two tap-water enemas, whereas children of 2 or more years of age passing normal stools will need a short period of dietary modification beforehand and some form of purge to clear the right colon.

Any dietary changes can be relatively minor and, in view of the short transit time to the right colon, need not be longer than 2 days.[3–5] On the first day indigestible foods (such as sweet corn and fiber-containing vegetables and fruits) are excluded or pureed, and on the afternoon before examination clear fluids and sloppy foods (fruit jelly, water-ice) are given as far as possible. It is unnecessary to starve before examination (if performed without anesthesia), and small amounts of sweet drinks will keep the child content without overstimulating the small intestine and refilling the right colon.

The purge to be used is to some extent a matter of personal preference. Senna syrup[7,10] has the virtue of tasting good and being effective and is easily adjusted in dose (1 ml/kg body weight). Other active agents such as bisacodyl and castor oil are equally effective but unpopular. Magnesium sulphate[3] is unpleasant to take and often ineffective because given in inadequate quantities. Magnesium citrate[4] is pleasant tasting but too gentle. (If a purge/magnesium citrate mixture (Picolax) is used, enemas can be avoided.). These purges take between 1 and 6 hours to work and are thus usually given in the late afternoon or early morning, depending on the time of procedure. About an hour beforehand one or two enemas are given; a 50-ml phosphate enema may be enough in babies, but a much larger volume (200–1500 ml of tap-water or saline) can be accommodated in the colon of older children. A competent and motivated nurse is needed to ensure that the proximal colon is reached and that the subsequent enema returns are clear. "Wash-outs" in which small volumes are run in and out of the distal colon will not clean the proximal colon for the purposes of total colonoscopy.

In children over about 5–6 years of age who are able to cooperate, one of the oral lavage[13] methods can be used, which avoids the need for enemas and requires only a short period of dieting. Mannitol (500 ml of a 10 percent solution) followed by large quantities of any clear fluid produces diarrhea within an hour, and colonoscopy should be possible 4 hours after administration. The solution should be drunk slowly; the chance of small intestinal distention with vomiting may be reduced by giving metoclopramide (10 mg) beforehand. The possibility of dehydration must be remembered in small or ill children. Mannitol, being a sugar, will result in bacterial fermentation to form hydrogen and should not be given before polypectomies. Drinking a flavored isotonic saline solution (2–4 liters) or using the gastric tube lavage technique (3–10 liters) achieves the same results, but drinking a large volume voluntarily or tolerating an intranasal tube may create problems. All the oral lavage techniques result in a considerable fluid residue in the colon that will slightly slow the procedure.

Sedation

The world literature shows a large number of centers often using general anesthesia for pediatric colonoscopy,[1,3–7,12,14–16] presumably because the authors are surgeons who assume that anesthesia is necessary and have no difficulty in arranging for an anesthetist. There are a number of reports from other centers, mostly from physicians who do not employ anesthesia[2,10,17,18]; we feel most strongly that this is the correct approach.

Quite apart from the not insignificant hazards of anesthesia, rendering the child senseless means that the endoscopist is deprived of the extremely useful warning sign of pain. Once the instrument has passed per anus there is no pain unless the colon is being overdistended by excessive insufflation or the colon and its attachments stretched by forceful looping of the instrument. A straightened instrument passing through the colon is painless, and the average colonoscopy should cause no more pain than the average visit to the dentist. On the other hand, it is possible to be clumsy with the instrument, which under anesthesia can result in damage to the colon, whereas a similar maneuver performed under sedation will be seen (and heard) to be cruel to the child. Equally, during electrosurgical polypectomy any pain experienced means that the serosal aspect of the bowel is being heated and full-thickness damage is imminent. Colonoscopy will only have a really useful role in pediatric practice if it can be frequently and easily used, often on an out-patient basis—a further reason to avoid thinking of colonoscopy as a major procedure requiring anesthesia.

On the other hand, intubation of any kind is an invasion of the body, feared, resented, and ill-remembered by any patient except a baby; some sedation is, therefore, desirable to allay fear, raise the pain threshold, and induce a degree of amnesia for the event. Babies up to 1 year old are quickly examined with a suitable instrument and not disturbed by fears or memory; they, therefore, may need no sedation. Above 1–2 years of age apprehension about the procedure is often the worst part of it. Suitable explanation and showing a soft rubber catheter of similar diameter to the instrument may be reassuring. The amount of sedation used can be much reduced by performing the examination in familiar or unfrightening surroundings.

Fibersigmoidoscopy with a pediatric instrument on a small trolley at the bedside should be no more traumatic than digital examination and might be managed without any sedation at all. For longer procedures, especially in the foreign territory of an endoscopy room, premedication 1–2 hours beforehand is essential. Oral (or rectal) medication with tranquilizing agents such as chloral or vallergan or intramuscular chlorpromazine (1 mg/kg) or pethidine (1–2 mg/kg) should render the child relaxed, slightly drowsy but cooperative on arrival for the examination. Thereafter an intravenous sedative/analgesic combination is used, the agents and dosage being variable, an experienced endoscopist with a good relationship and a few candies needing a relatively low dose so that the patient is less sedated afterwards. Diazepam has advantageous amnestic effects but may make children uncontrollable, whereas pethidine (or meperidine) is a very good tranquilizer as well as analgesic, reversible afterwards by naloxone, but does not cause amnesia. The combination of a low dose of diazepam and a higher dose of pethidine, given slowly and titrated to some extent according to drowsiness, has a maximal effect for the 2 minutes needed to pass through the sigmoid colon, the child being only mildly drowsy by the end of the procedure. Intravenous naloxone (0.2 mg) works within 20–30 seconds in reversing the effect of the pethidine if the child is oversedated.

Antispasmodic agents such as hyoscine-*N*-butyl bromide (10–20 mg IV) or glucagon (0.25–0.5 mg IV) are occasionally useful to ensure a good view in the presence of spasm, a relatively unusual problem because of the spasmolytic properties of the sedatives already administered.

Indications

In pediatric practice, as has already been indicated, the usefulness of colonoscopy is increased by the importance of early diagnosis and the relative difficulty of obtaining satisfactory barium enema pictures and biopsy specimens. Almost any patient with abdominal symptoms might have fibersigmoidoscopy or limited colonoscopy, but a clearer idea is needed about when total colonoscopy is indicated.

Bleeding

Bleeding is a particularly strong indication for colonoscopy, often as a primary procedure, although the results are frequently negative. The fibercolonoscope does not replace careful anal inspection or palpation for local pathologic conditions, such as fissure, but above the anus the advantage of color view and the biopsy/polypectomy potential of the endoscope make it much more likely to be rewarding than the barium enema. If total colonoscopy proves difficult the proximal colon can be rechecked immediately afterward on barium enema while the colon is clean, providing that any air is aspirated or carbon dioxide (rapidly absorbed) insufflation used so that the colon is left undistended for the radiologist. The whole colon should normally be examined, since juvenile polyps (the commonest cause of colonic bleeding in childhood) may exist throughout the colon (see Figure 25, p. vi). When there is a history of substantial bleeding and both colonoscopy and gastroduodenoscopy prove normal, the diagnosis of Meckel's diverticulum is overwhelmingly likely.

Anemia

Anemia is usually investigated in the context of suspected inflammatory bowel disease or known hemangiomas or hamartomatous polyposis.

Diarrhea

Diarrhea of over 1 week's duration merits at least limited colonoscopy, particularly if accompanied by bleeding to suggest primarily colonic origin. The cause may be infective, allergic, or inflammatory, and histological and microbiological assessment as well as naked eye opinion may be useful in differential diagnosis.

Pain

Pain alone is a relatively unrewarding indication, the diagnosis usually proving to be that of a functional disorder with normal colonoscopy. In children with right-sided abdominal pain there may be doubt on x-ray in differentiation between abnormality of the terminal ileum and nodular lymphoid hyperplasia. Normal findings on colonoscopy may give powerful reassurance to worried parents or doctors managing a chronic problem.

Inflammatory Bowel Disease

Inflammatory bowel disease, suspected or known, can be most accurately assessed at colonoscopy. Very limited colonoscopy, with little or no preparation or sedation, can be invaluable in followup to assess response to treatment. Questionable recurrences or unexplained symptoms (such as pain associated with mild disease) may be worth checking, since colitis patients can have unrelated functional bowel symptoms. It may be important to know the exact extent of inflammation in deciding on the correct treatment regimen; colonoscopy with biopsy is the most accurate means of achieving this and can provide biopsy diagnosis of right-sided or ileal disease with differential diagnosis from other forms of colitis such as tuberculosis or *Yersinia*.

X-Ray Abnormalities

X-ray abnormalities such as strictures or possible polyps are easily confirmed or excluded. Polyps of any size can normally be snared at colonoscopy at any site in the colon and surgery should never be required.

Screening Examination

Screening examination of members of at-risk families, as in adenomatous polyposis coli, is more easily and acccurately performed by limited colonoscopy than any other means. Biopsy evidence is essential to ensure that any lesions found are neoplastic polyps rather than hamartomatous lesions or lymphoid follicles. Multiple polypectomies are possible in patients with juvenile or Peutz-Jeghers polyposis.

Contraindications and Complications

The only contraindication to colonoscopy in children is the presence of features suggesting easy bowel perforation, such as radiological full-thickness ulceration, acute fistulation or toxic megacolon, or clinical signs of acute abdominal tenderness or peritonism.

The complication rate in diagnostic pediatric colonoscopy appears to be very low.[6] From adult experience it can be expected that occasional complication will arise relating to medication or sepsis in susceptible (immunodeficient or immunosuppressed) individuals as well as to instrument trauma. Traumatic effects are presumably rare because of the great elasticity of the childhood colon.

Polypectomy, however, alters the balance; juvenile polyps are frequently of large size and the colon is proportionately thinner than that of adults. The early pediatric colonoscopy literature showed a 5 percent incidence of bowel perforation during or after polypectomy,[3-5,15,19] and as series grow larger there may be an incidence of immediate or delayed (5–10 days) hemorrhage from the transected polyp stalks.

Colonoscopy Technique

In the pediatric age range, from the neonatal period to young adulthood, there is a considerable change in the characteristics of the colon, with consequent effects on instrumentation and technique. The least marked change is in anal or colonic diameter. Digital anorectal examination is possible at any age and the diameter of the instrument is only important because insertion of a narrower instrument is more comfortable and thinner instruments are more easily made flexible. Although the baby colon is shorter, it is, by virtue of being very elastic, relatively long in its sigmoid part, which can be pushed up to the diaphragm. The attachments of the baby colon are also freer, with a tendency for the descending colon in particular to be mobile on a mesocolon, resulting in awkward "reverse" looping (Figure 8-2), which may make total colonoscopy difficult. The general details of instrument-handling and intubational techniques are fully described elsewhere.[12]

The position of the child during colonoscopy is of little importance, babies and small children usually being examined on their backs, but older children often being more comfortable in the left lateral position. Shinya (in a personal communication) describes total colonoscopy of a baby being hugged by its mother. In small children it is essential that instrument handling is gentle and dexterous so as to pass through the sigmoid colon without looping; anything more than the slightest loop will cause acute angulation, with difficulty and pain in passing from the sigmoid to the de-

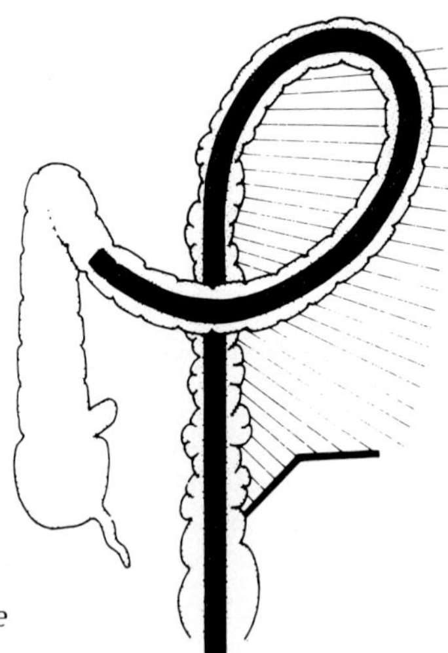

Figure 8-2. *"Reverse" looping at the splenic flexure due to a descending mesocolon.*

scending colon. Babies respond to overstretching of the sigmoid by becoming quiet, the first sign of shock. Gentle and coordinated technique with frequent withdrawal to keep the instrument straight rather than looped can only be achieved using "single-handed" manipulation, the endoscopist's left hand managing the controls and his right hand the instrument shaft. The assistant is occasionally useful to steady the instrument or to compress the lower abdomen to resist loop formation but is rarely needed to advance the instrument. Accurate steering is obviously also necessary and best practiced in the more capacious adult colon before starting pediatric examinations.

In the learning phase it is valuable to use fluoroscopy (image intensification) in a few cases, mainly to prove the tendency to looping and the importance of pulling back repeatedly to avoid or remove them. Fluoroscopy may also be useful in the unexpectedly difficult case or to localize a lesion when transillumination or instrument distance are inconclusive. Since few pediatric endoscopists are likely to acquire the large personal experience that their adult colleagues do, some reliance on fluoroscopy may be desirable, although it should be used as little as possible so as not to overirradiate either patient or instrument and so as to learn rapid empirical instrument technique. If the instrument can be kept pulled back and straight, passage into the descending colon is easy; manual pressure on the abdomen helps to pass round the splenic flexure without relooping. Once in the transverse colon it is easy to pass on to the cecum, using a combination of pull-back technique, air aspiration, and further manual compression of any unavoidable loops. Although it may be surprising to reach the cecum with only 30–40 cm of a straightened instrument, seeing fecal residue at the pole and transillumination at the right iliac fossa confirms the tip position. Total colonoscopy is possible in over 90 percent of children without undue difficulties. The ileocecal valve varies in appearance but is always 3–4 cm distal to the cecal pole, usually being seen as a soft, dimpled protuberance. Hooking the tip into the center of this bulge or fold, pulling back, and insufflating will almost always allow the tip to be passed for at least 5–25 cm into the ileum. If the colonoscope is still looped and is, therefore, at a mechanical disadvantage, or if the valve is strictured by inflammation, passage may be impossible; even so, the visible inner margin of the valve lip being composed of small intestinal mucosa, it will usually be ulcerated if the ileum is abnormal, and vice versa.

Although limited colonoscopy is quick and easy, total colonoscopy and ileoscopy can sometimes be traumatic or impossible, especially in older children. If this is so the procedure should be abandoned for referral, if clinically indicated, to an experienced adult endoscopist. Unless the difficulty is due to adhesions, by a combination of maneuvring and use of different instruments or accessories such as the stiffening overtube, the examination can almost always be successful.

Polypectomy and Electrosurgical Techniques

The techniques of polypectomy and electrosurgery in pediatric colonoscopy are comparable in all respects to those employed in adult endoscopy and very fully described elsewhere.[12] Certain basic principles and points, however, deserve repetition. Polypectomy with electrosurgery in conscious patients is completely safe and painless, since the high-frequency current used does not shock. Neither inside nor at the patient plate should any sensation be felt. When using the polypectomy snare or the insulated hot-biopsy forceps for electrocoagulation, some dexterity is needed to manipulate the instrument tip so as to position the accessory accurately. The sharp bends of the colon and the large size of some polyps may mean that there is very poor view of what is happening, which can make it difficult to judge if the lesion is properly caught and then to see when it is securely electrocoagulated. Although in theory the polyp is held into the center of the lumen, avoiding contact with the opposite bowel wall, the 2-cm diameter of many juvenile polyps makes this quite impossible, with the result that current spread away from the stalk makes heating and coagulation more difficult (Figure 8-3). A useful trick for the management of large and thick-stalked polyps in the sigmoid colon is that of snare-loop intussusception,[20] in which the polyp is first snared endoscopically and the child then briefly anesthetized for full relaxation, the polyp being pulled down to the anus for removal and ligation by local surgical means.

Other large polyps should usually only be tackled with the assistance of an experienced adult endoscopist aware of the potential danger of perforation of a thin childhood colon. If large polyps are known to be present it is desirable to have blood available and probably to perform coagulation studies, for the feeding vessels in the stalk may be substantial with the possibility of major hemorrhage. The child can be discharged the day after polypectomy, for there have not (as yet) been reports of secondary or delayed hemorrhage in children. Such delayed hemorrhages in adults normally stop spontaneously.

Whereas large polyps require some care, small polyps and hemangiomas are extremely easily and rapidly coagulated. Because childhood polyps are almost invariably hamartomatous and without neoplastic potential (except in adenomatous polyposis coli) it may be justifiable to remove several or numerous polyps but only to retrieve or wash out afterward a representative number for histologic examination.

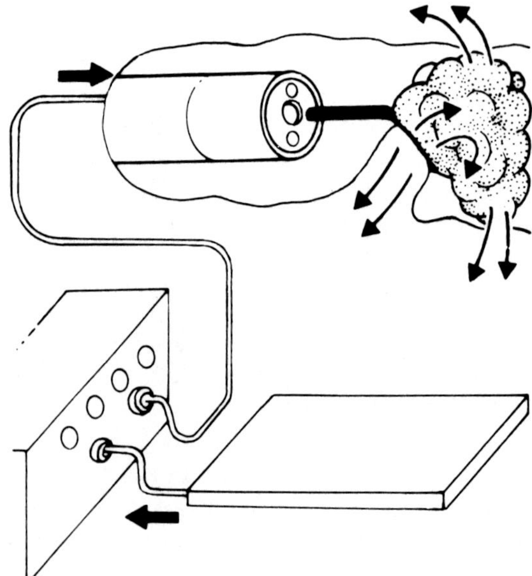

Figure 8-3. *Contact by a large polyp head with the bowel wall results in current flow away from the polyp stalk and inefficient stalk electrocoagulation.*

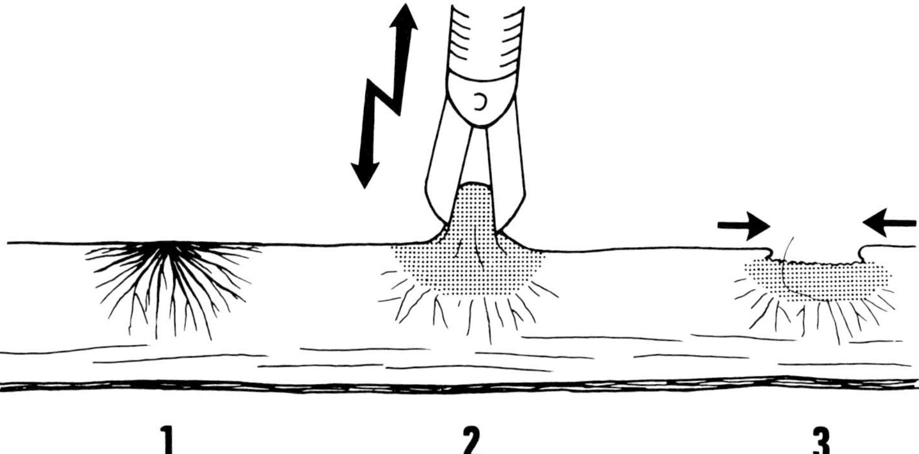

Figure 8-4. *Diagrammatic representation of the "hot-biopsy" technique for safe electrocoagulation and subsequent re-epithelialization over a small telangiectasis.*

Large, diffuse hemangiomas are unsuited to electrosurgery and probably even to laser photocoagulation, since the feeding vessels are extracolonic so that recurrence is inevitable. Small hemangiomas require only brief electrocoagulation, pulling up with the hot-biopsy forceps[23,29] to reduce the chance of full-thickness damage, resulting in a surprisingly large ulcer. Presumably this re-epithelializes (Figure 8-4) over any remaining vascular lesion. Larger, cavernous hemangiomas, such as the "blue rubber bleb nevus" syndrome, can be endoscopically sclerosed using the retractable injection needle to infiltrate ethanolamine oleate.

The Clinical Yield of Colonoscopy

Many of the gains of colonoscopy have been mentioned above, based on a combined experience from our personal series of over 2,000 pediatric colonoscopies. The available literature on pediatric colonoscopy is extremely scant and clearly suggests that the application of colonoscopy to pediatric gastroenterology has been slow in evolution, partly because specially built pediatric colonoscopes have not been commercially available. While adult colonoscopes can be used, they feel very clumsy in the bowel of a small child, whereas some of the slim and more flexible prototype instruments of which we have experience are gentler to insert and easier to use. Not surprisingly, pediatricians have tended so far to rely on adult endoscopists for help and instrumentation.[4,10] Perhaps when pediatricians are able to buy their own instruments and have a commitment to use them the practicality of colonoscopy, its immediate yield, the photographs, biopsies, and therapeutic dividends in the first few patients examined will result in the same avalanche of enthusiasm for colonoscopy that has occurred in adult gastroenterology.

Several authors have stressed the great usefulness of colonoscopy in overt or occult bleeding. Habr-Gama et al.[3] found rectal bleeding to be their main indication for colonoscopy in a series of 53 examinations. When a diagnosis was made it was of polyps and the results of barium enema were found to be so inferior that they recommend colonoscopy as the screening procedure of choice in children with continued or profuse bleeding. Holgerson, Mossberg, and Miller[4] consider that barium enema should precede colonoscopy in bleeding patients, although x-ray was positive in only two of several conoloscopically diagnosed children, missing the diagnosis in two shown by colonoscopy to have acute colitis and three shown to have polyps. The results of all series are enormously affected by clinical case selection of those patients examined, but colonoscopy obviously makes a major contribution as potential management for any bleeding patient.

Some of the hemangiomas seen earlier in our series were unsuitable for electrocoagulation, although this should have been possible for the 2 × 3 cm lesion described by Skovgaard and Sorensen[21] and the three cases reported by Fisher, Harrison; and Adkins.[14] The place of laser photocoagulation in pediatric practice is conjectural, but the controlled, very superficial coagulation possible with the argon laser has attractions. Management with local electrocoagulation[23] or injection sclerotherapy (1 ml ethanolamine) has been possible and effective in several patients in our series with multiple cavernous hemangiomas (blue rubber bleb nevus syndrome).

It is a truism to say that early diagnosis of diarrheal conditions in childhood is of the greatest importance, and in our personal series the major single clinical indication has been suspected inflammatory bowel disease, whether infective or nonspecific. Diarrhea unresolved after a week or more, even when probably infective in origin, may usefully be investigated by limited colonoscopy; often the presentation of our cases has been of children with progressive ill health and a history of months of fruitless investigation by conventional means at other hospitals.

The diagnosis of mild Crohn's disease in particular presents great difficulties for assessment either by rectal biopsy (because of frequent sparing of the rectum) or barium enema (because the aphthoid ulcers of the earlier stages of the disease may be scattered and superficial). There is also an understandable reluctance on the part of paediatricians to commit a child to treatment with "heavy" medication such as corticosteroids or immunosuppressants without definite evidence. For this purpose the endoscopic view of a friable and bleeding or superficially ulcerated mucosa is much more convincing than a doubtful x-ray change[24,25] even if the biopsies are not always diagnostic, which, as Habr-Gama et al.[3] have pointed out, is frequently the case. Even in the presence of characteristic small or discrete apthoid ulcers of Crohn's disease, set in the normal background mucosa, we have found only a 25 percent yield of diagnostic granulomata [10] In many of the remaining cases an experienced pathologist is, however, been able to say that the chronic inflammatory process was "unlike ulcerative colitis and more suggestive of Crohn's disease," because of the patchy nature of the abnormality and relative preservation of the goblet cell population. Biopsies in suspected Crohn's disease are taken both at the margin of the smallest lesion seen and in the intervening normal mucosa so as to demonstrate to the pathologist the endoscopically obvious patchiness (Figure 8-5). Even in definite cases of amebic colitis or other infections small biopsies may not be diagnostic, although the pathologist can say from the relative excess of acute inflammatory cells (polymorphs and eosinophils) that an infective cause is likely.

In about 10 percent of cases, certain differential diagnoses between the various specific and nonspecific causes of inflammatory bowel disease may be impossible. It is obviously wise in all cases to perform prior stool culture for *Shigella, Salmonella Yersinia* and *Campylobacter.* Sometimes culture of colonoscopic biopsies will give a result when conventional stool culture techniques have failed. Often serology

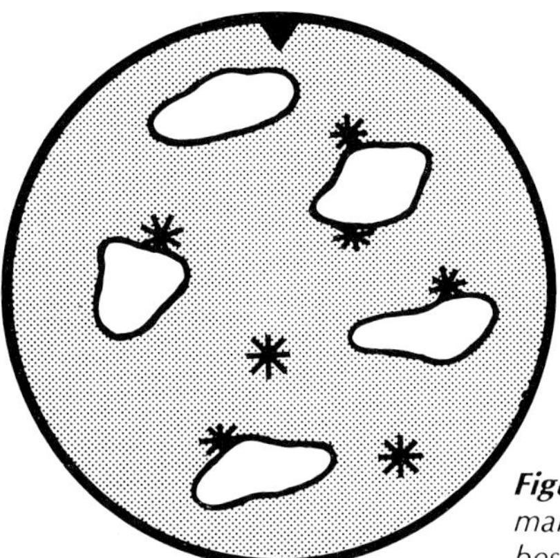

Figure 8-5. *Six to eight biopsies taken both at the margins and between small Crohn's ulcers give the best chance of histopathologic confirmation.*

is indicated to exclude amebiasis or *Yersinia,* although the latter is apparently rare outside Belgium.

Ulcerative colitis, as a specifically epithelial condition, is more satisfactorily diagnosed on colonoscopic biopsies, sometimes when the endoscopic abnormality is very slight and the x-ray appearances normal. Habr-Gama et al.[3] diagnosed ulcerative colitis in two children with a normal barium enema study and we have experience of a number of cases of both ulcerative and Crohn's colitis where extensive mild inflammatory change, sometimes affecting the whole colon, was missed on barium enema. In all such patients there was a clinical suspicion of inflammatory disease on the basis of suggestive features in the history, together with either anemia or a raised sedimentation rate. As a result, we now favor colonoscopy as part of the initial workup of possible inflammatory disease, sometimes without performing barium enema. At least five or six biopsies are taken throughout the colon to demonstrate the extent of inflammatory process in ulcerative colitis, which often extends somewhat further on microscopy than is apparent endosciopically. The biopsies taken at colonoscopy are so small that there is no contraindication to performing a barium enema on the prepared colon afterwards, whereas obviously a barium-filled colon makes endoscopy impossible. In a few cases, it has been possible merely to insufflate air to distend the colon after colonoscopy and then to take an air film to demonstrate the colon outline on a plain film.

Except in the case of adenomatous polyposis coli, when there will normally be a family history, polyps in childhood are hamartomatous and removed only to prevent bleeding and anemia. In patients with the Peutz-Jeghers syndrome, prophylactic gastroscopy and colonoscopy (top and tail endoscopy) are possible in a single session so as to remove any larger polyps, sometimes amounting to 15 or 20 polyps in all; often there will be a number of smaller polyps left in situ which may disappear by the time of further examination 2–3 years later. These polyps and the juvenile hamartomas, of which three or four greater than 2-cm examples may be found throughout the colon of small children,[2,11,16,17] are characterized by relatively thin stalks. Even large diameter polyps in childhood should, therefore, be amendable to endoscopic management; one of our patients had a 5-cm-diameter juvenile polyp that appeared sessile radiologically but proved to be on a 5-mm stalk. One 2-year-old had a 3.5-cm polyp in the proximal sigmoid colon removed at the anus after snare-loop intussusception, since the stalk appeared relatively thick with potential danger of either hemorrhage or bowel wall damage on overcoagulation. Perforations have been reported in four cases[3–5,15] in the reported series of pediatric polypectomies,[3–5,9,10,15–17] giving a 1 percent incidence in childhood compared to the 0.34 percent perforation rate in adult polypectomies reported by Fruhmorgen[22] and personal experience of 0.05 percent perforation in 2,000 adult polypectomies. In addition, Gleason et al.[17] describe a child with postpolypectomy pain and fever, indicating a full-thickness burn with serosal involvement, nonoperatively managed. Adult experience would suggest that, in the presence of a completely clean colon and the absence of bleeding, many of even the frank perforations can be successfully managed nonoperatively under antibiotic cover.

Extra care is obviously needed during pediatric polypectomy. Since hemorrhage has *not* been reported (Fruhmorgen[22] found a 2 percent adult hemorrhage rate), it is presumably preferable to use a minimum of electrocoagulation for pediatric polypectomy and to apply the snare at the apex of the stalk; if bleeding does occur this site should make it easy to resnare and mechanically strangle the bleeding stalk for 15–20 minutes, by which time coagulation should have occurred.

Habr-Gama et al.[3] remark on the relative inaccuracy of x-rays for identification of polyps, both because of false-positives (because of poor bowel preparation) and missed lesions. Juvenile polyps are well known to autoamputate[22] and we have experience in several cases of finding at endoscopy only the residual polyp stalk, whereas the polyp head could be seen on the preceding x-ray. Nelson et al.[27] mention the importance, in any patient known to have one or more polyps, of performing total colonscopy because of the relatively high incidence of juvenile polyps in the proximal colon.

The overall experience of pediatric colonscopy is still too small to know what the potential may be for particular techniques or diagnostic uses that relate only to childhood. Willital[28] has, for instance, used the colonoscope for preoperative placement of magnetic slugs in the management of imperforate anus. Removal of ingested foreign bodies is likely to be of some importance, the only case in our series having been an impacted pin, successfully extracted. Lymphoid hyperplasia of the colon or terminal ileum is often a normal finding, but we have seen a superficially similar appearance in a unique case of lipoid polyposis. Childhood conditions such as Schönlein-Henoch purpura may be seen affecting the colon, and doubtless other colonic manifestations of immunological and allergic disturbances will be described. Georgraphic variation and case selection can produce as common diagnoses in some series (e.g., schistosomal polyps by Habr-Gama et al.) conditions that are rare or nonexistent in others.

Conclusion

Pediatric colonoscopy is a practical and rewarding procedure in certain circumstances, especially for bleeding or suspected inflammatory bowel. disease. The childhood colon is relatively easy to prepare and the examination well tolerated under sedation alone. Pediatric gastroenterologist and gastrointestinal surgeons should seriously consider undertaking at least limited colonoscopy as a routine procedure in the ward or outpatient clinic. Difficult total colonoscopies and, for the time being, polypectomies should be left for an experienced endoscopist.

References

1. Burdelski M: Endoscopy in paediatric gastroenterology. Eur J Pediatr 128:33–39, 1978
2. Cadranel S, Rodesch P, Peeters, JP, et al: Fiber-endoscopy of the gastrointestinal tract in children. Am J Dis Child 131:41; 1977
3. Habr-Gama A, Alves AA, Gama-Rodriques JJ: Paediatric colonoscopy. Dis Colon Rectum 22:530–535, 1979
4. Holgerson LO, Mossberg SM, Miller RE: Colonoscopy for rectal bleeding in childhood. J Pediatr Surg 13:83 –85, 1978
5. Liebman WM: Fibreoptic endoscopy of the gastrointestinal tract in infants and children. Am J Gastroenterol 68:452–455, 1977
6. Livstone EM, Cohen GM, Troncale FJ, et al: Diastatic serosal lacerations: an unrecognised complication of colonoscopy. Gastroenterology 67:1245–1247, 1974
7. Lux G, Rosch W, Phillip J, et al: Gastrointestinal fibreoptic endoscopy in paediatric patients and juveniles. Endoscopy 10:158–163, 1978
8. Plucnar J: Colonoscopy in infancy and childhood with special regard to patient preparation and examination technique. Endoscopy 13:14–18, 1981
9. Rodesch P, Cadranel S, Peeters JP, et al: Colonic endoscopy in children. Acta Paediatr Belg 29(3): 181–184, 1976
10. Williams CB, Laage NJ, Campbell CA, et al: Total colonoscopy in children. Child 57:49–53, 1982
11. Cremer M, Peeters JP, Emonts P, et al: Fiberendoscopy of the gastrointestinal tract in children—experience with newly designed fibrescopes. Endoscopy 6:186–189, 1974
12. Cotton PB, Williams CB: Practical Gastrointestinal Endoscopy. Oxford, Blackwell, 1980
13. Levy AG, Benson JW, Hewlett EL, et al: Saline lavage. Lancet 70:157–166, 1976
14. Fisher SE, Harrison M, Adkins JC: Colonoscopic diagnosis of vascular abnormalities in children. 18:299–303, 1979
15. Gans SL, Ament M, Christie DL, et al: Paediatric endoscopy with flexible fibrescopes. J Pediatr Surg 10:375–380, 1975
16. King JF, Smith GE: Endoscopic removal of recurrent juvenile polyps in a six year old. Gastroenterology 66A:815, 1974
17. Gleason WA, Goldstein PD, Shatz BA, et al: Colonoscopic removal of juvenile polyps. J Pediatr Surg 10:519–521, 1975
18. Graham DY: Value of fibreoptic gastrointestinal endoscopy in infants and childhood. South Med J 71:558–560, 1978
19. Daum, F, Zucker P, Boley SJ, et al: Colonscopic polypectomy in children. Am J Dis Child 1977
20. Gillespie PE, Nicholls RJ, Thomson JP, et al: Snare polypectomy by sigmoid-rectal intussusception: NZ Med J 1:1395, 1978
21. Skovgaard S, Sorensen FH: Bleeding haemangioma of the colon diagnosed by colonoscopy. J Pediatr Surg 11:83–84, 1976
22. Fruhmorgen P, Demling L: Complications of diagnostic and therapeutic colonoscopy in the Federal Republic of Germany. Endoscopy 11:146, 1979
23. Williams CB: Diathermy-biopsy—a technique for the endoscopic management of small polyps. Endoscopy 5:215–218, 1973
24. Burdelski M, Huchzermeyer H, Lucking T, et al: Endoscopic findings in children with Crohn's disease. Acta Paediatr Belg 30:193–199, 1977
25. Mougenot JF, Mathe JC, Neueschwander S, et al: Endoscopic features of Crohn's disease in children. Acta Paediatr Belg 3:200–203, 1977
26. Douglas JR, Campbell CA, Salisbury DM; Colonoscopic polypectomy in children Br Med J 281:1386–1387, 1981
27. Nelson EN, Rodgers BM, Zawatzky L: Endoscopic appearance of autoamputated polyps in juvenile polyposis coli. J Pediatr Surg 12: 773–6 1978
28. Willital A H: Significance of paediatric endoscopy. Endoscopy 10:153–157, 1978
29. Rogers BHG: Endoscopic diagnosis and therapy of mucosal vascular abnormalties. Gastrointest Endoc 26:134–138, 1980

Urologic Endoscopy

CHAPTER 9

W. Hardy Hendren

Endoscopy is a vital part of the armamentarium in treating disorders of the urinary tract in infants and children. The urinary tract is especially well suited to precise anatomic and pathologic assessment by combining the modalities of modern radiographic techniques with direct-vision endoscopy. There should be no mystique surrounding urologic endoscopy in infants and children. A surgeon with reasonable dexterity and expertise in endoscopy of other systems, such as esophagoscopy and bronchoscopy, can become proficient in urologic endoscopy as well. Suitable equipment is needed, together with a population of patients who require study. In this chapter are covered some essentials and "tricks" that we have found useful in the past 25 years.

Endoscopy findings can often affect the decision whether to operate or not. We believe, therefore, that cystoscopy should be a routine measure in evaluation of the pediatric urinary tract. Urinary tract screening should never consist of just an intravenous pyelogram. If there are urologic symptoms, particularly infection, adequate workup should include intravenous pyelography, voiding cystourethrography, and usually cystourethroscopy. Much useful information can be obtained during cystoscopy. In addition to inspecting the interior of the bladder, observation should also include the full length of urethra and the vagina too in female patients.

General anesthesia is always used for urologic endoscopy in children. Diagnostic cystoscopy is done on a transient admission basis. The patient comes to the hospital early with an empty stomach. Blood hemoglobin is determined previously. After a physical examination, inhalation anesthesia is administered by mask for the procedure. The child is generally discharged by late morning. Although it is nice to have a special endoscopy suite available, with an endoscopy operating table, built in x-ray equipment, and so forth, that is by no means imperative. We routinely perform our endoscopic procedures on an ordinary operating table in lithotomy position, in the same operating room that will be used for an open procedure if one is to be needed, generally under the same anesthesia. Adequate x-ray films can be obtained using portable x-ray machines, although that does not allow fluoroscopy. This has not proved to be disadvantageous in recent years, with more use of antegrade, perfusion studies in the conscious patient in the radiology department prior to endoscopy to observe ureteral emptying, peristalsis, and so on.

Scrupulous aseptic technique should be practiced during cystoscopy. It is an invasive procedure in which bacteria can be introduced directly into the urinary tract by careless technique. The anus should be suitably draped from the operative field. The eyepiece of the endoscope is contaminated at the outset. Those handling the instrument must thus take that into account. I have seen on many occasions endoscopists contaminating their fingertips on the eyepiece and then passing retrograde catheters into the kidney with unsterile fingers. Good surgical technique can minimize introduction of infection by the surgeon. Endoscopy should be postponed whenever possible in patients with active acute infection. A urine sample is collected for culture and sensitivities during cystoscopy. Some patients will prove to have significant bacilluria despite absence of symptoms. Occasionally a patient will develop high fever following endoscopy, especially if retrograde pyelography has been performed. The culture with antibiotic sensitivities taken at the time of the endoscopic procedure will prove useful in guiding treatment.

Equipment

Until about 15 years ago cystoscopy in infants and children using relatively large incandescent endoscopes was at best crude, as compared to what can be done today. The advent of the Hopkins rod lens system with fiberoptic illumination transformed pediatric endoscopy of all types into a precise diagnostic modality, with instruments sufficiently miniaturized to make these procedures practical in even the smallest infants.[1]

The basic cystoscopy setup we use routinely is shown in Figure 9-1. It includes solutions and sponges to prepare the skin, towel clips to hold drapes, mineral oil to lubricate instruments, a culture tube, a probe, scissors, and necessary cords and tubing. It includes pediatric urethral sounds to pass gently in males to calibrate the size of the urethra before passing the endoscope, and bougie à boules to pass in females to calibrate urethral size. The telescopes and sheaths on the table depend on the age and size of the patient. Pediatric endoscopes of great precision and using fiberoptic illumination are now available from Karl Storz, Richard Wolf, ACMI, and several other firms. Special additional items such as ureteral catheters are added to the table as needed.

A pediatric resectoscope should be part of the instrument armamentarium, although we seldom use it (Figure 9-2). On those few occasions where this instrument is employed it is usually to obtain a biopsy specimen from the bladder wall.

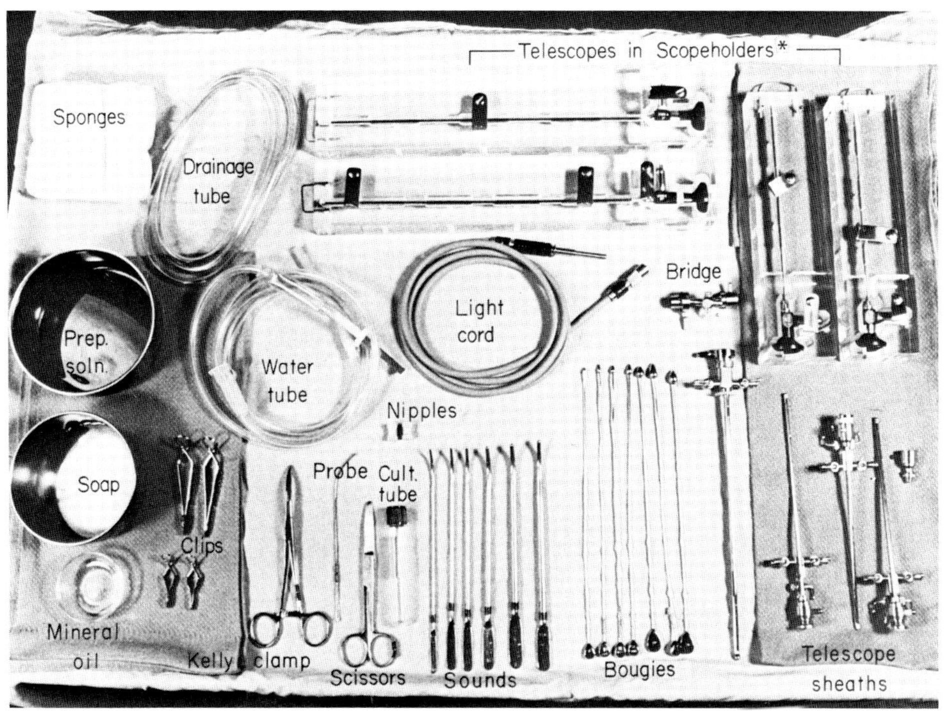

Figure 9-1. *Basic cystoscopy table setup. Special additional equipment such as ureteral catheters or instruments for meatotomy are added when needed. (Autoclavable telescope holders are available from Scopeholder Inc., P.O. Box 14 SHS, Duxbury, Massachusetts 02332.)*

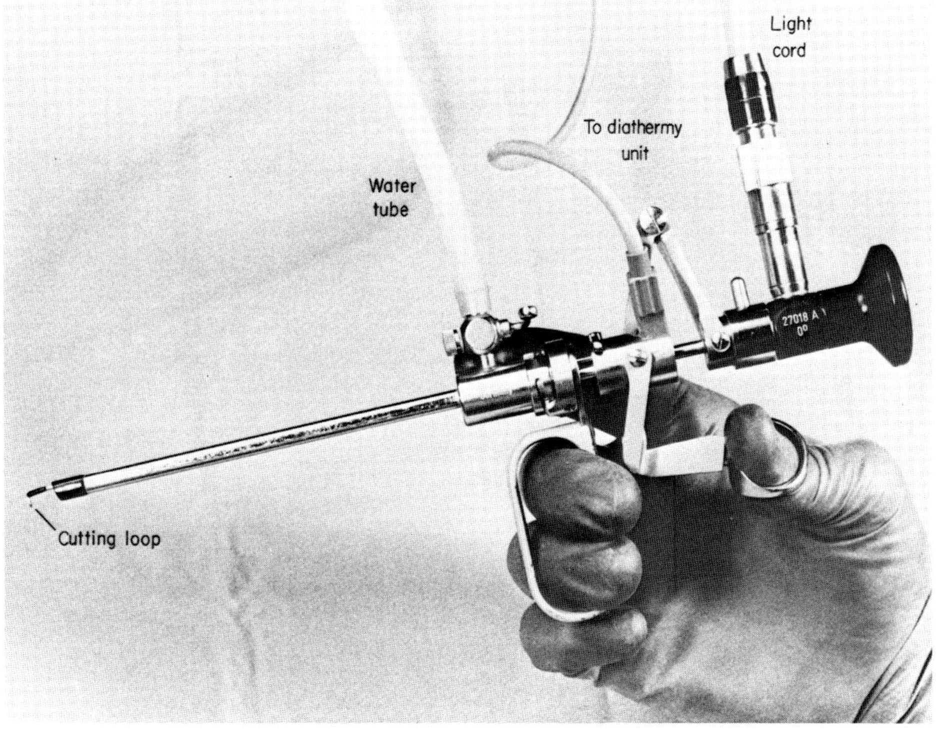

Figure 9-2. *Storz pediatric resectoscope.*

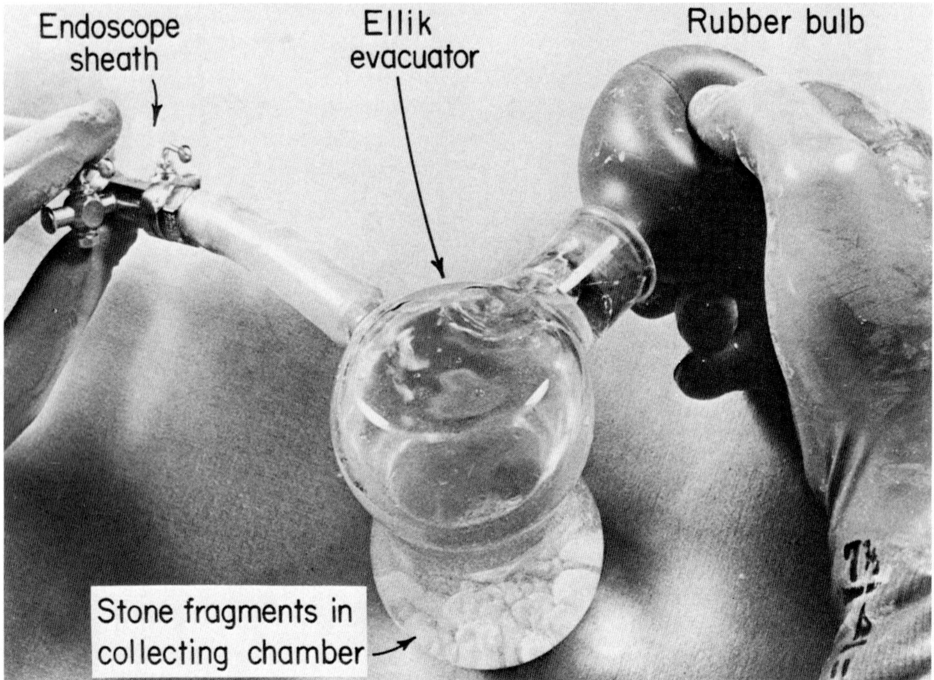

Figure 9-3. *Ellik evacuator to wash blood clot or small stone particles from bladder.*

The most frequent indication for an endoscopic cutting procedure in a child is transurethral resection of urethral valves. The resectoscope is *not* the best way to do that (see later section on Urethral Valves).

An Ellik evacuator is useful for washing out blood clots or stone fragments from the bladder (Figure 9-3). It is filled with solution and attached to the end of the panendoscope sheath. Intermittently squeezing and releasing its rubber bulb results in a brisk flow of water from the instrument to the bladder and back. Blood clots or stone fragments that come back with the irrigating solution settle in the collecting bowl of the evacuator. It can avert the need for bladder exploration for removal of clots or small stone fragments.

A Fogarty balloon embolectomy catheter can be useful in certain lower urinary tract operations. For example, in some very masculinized females with the adrenogenital syndrome the vagina enters the urethra at the level of the verumontanum.[2] Through the panendoscope a Fogarty embolectomy catheter can be passed into the vagina, inflating the balloon with air. This facilitates localization of the vaginal-urethral junction at operation, minimizing the dissection needed.

Technique for Instrumentation

Instrumentation of female patients, whose urethra is relatively short and straight, requires little expertise. Bougies of increasing size are passed to assess the caliber of the meatus, external sphincter, and bladder neck. A panendoscope of appropriate size is then passed, first dilating the urethra with sounds if that is necessary.

Endoscopy in the male requires much more finesse. If it is done poorly serious complications can result. The technique for passing a sound or a panendoscope is shown in Figure 9-4. With the penis on gentle traction, a well-lubricated instrument of appropriate size is passed straight in toward the bulbous urethra. The instrument is then depressed about 90° until it slides easily through the prostatic urethra, over the bladder neck, and into the bladder. An appropriately small instrument should be used. One that is too large traumatizes the delicate mucosa; this can result in stricture. An instrument must never be forced, lest it puncture the delicate urethral wall, making a false passage. If there is any resistance on passing an instrument, it should be done under direct vision, looking in through the telescope as it is being advanced (see also later remarks on urethral stricture).

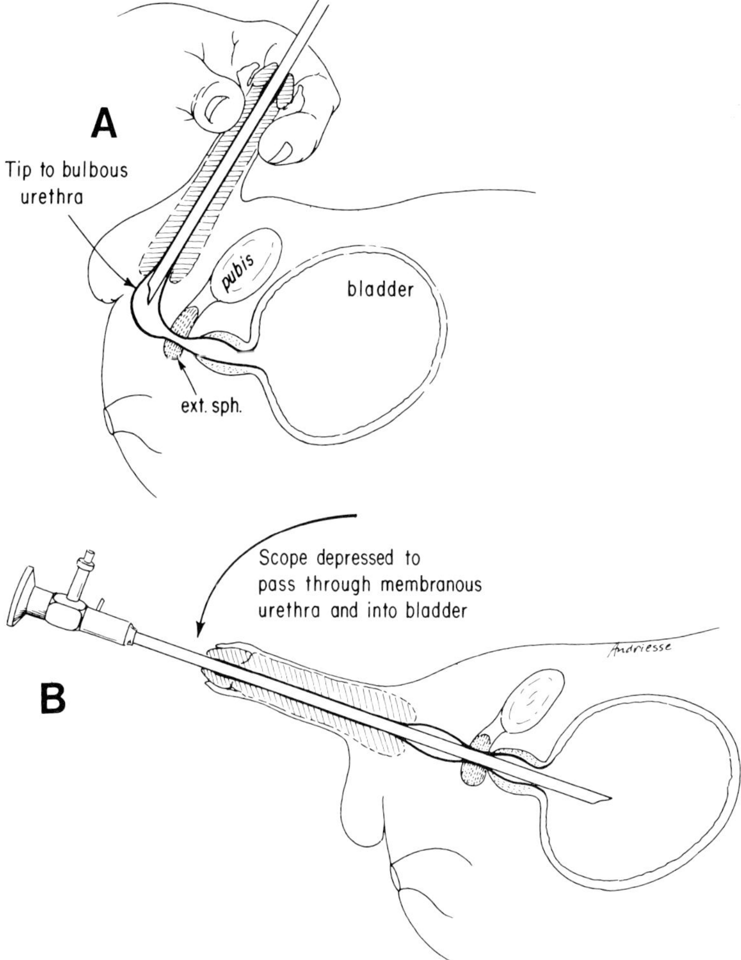

Figure 9-4. *Technique for instrumentation of male. (A) Instrument is passed gently to bulbous urethra, where urethra takes right-angle turn before passing through external sphincter beneath pubic symphysis. (B) Instrument is depressed downward and advanced without resistance into the bladder. If this right-angle turn in the urethra is instrumented too forcefully the posterior wall of the bulbous urethra can be perforated, causing a false passage between the urethra and the anterior wall of the rectum.*

It is an invitation to disaster to attempt endoscopy on a small male without miniaturized equipment. Figure 9-5 shows two of the most popular infant endoscopes, both only 8 F caliber. They will pass readily into the small urethra of most male infants weighing as little as 5–6 pounds. Formerly the instrument used for young males was the incandescent McCarthy panendoscope, which was much larger. Occasionally a male infant will not accept an 8 F scope. In this case one can perform perineal urethrostomy, shown in Figure 9-6. This bypasses the smaller penile urethra, entering directly into the bulbous urethra. This permits visualization of the urethra proximal to that point, generally for the problem of urethral valves. There should be no injury if the procedure is done skillfully. In actual practice we have not needed to use perineal urethrostomy for vizualizing the urethra in a male during the past 5 years. An especially small infant's urethra can be viewed by filling the bladder with an infant feeding tube and passing the Storz telescope without its sheath, while compressing the bladder to distend the urethra with fluid (see also the section on Urethral Valves).

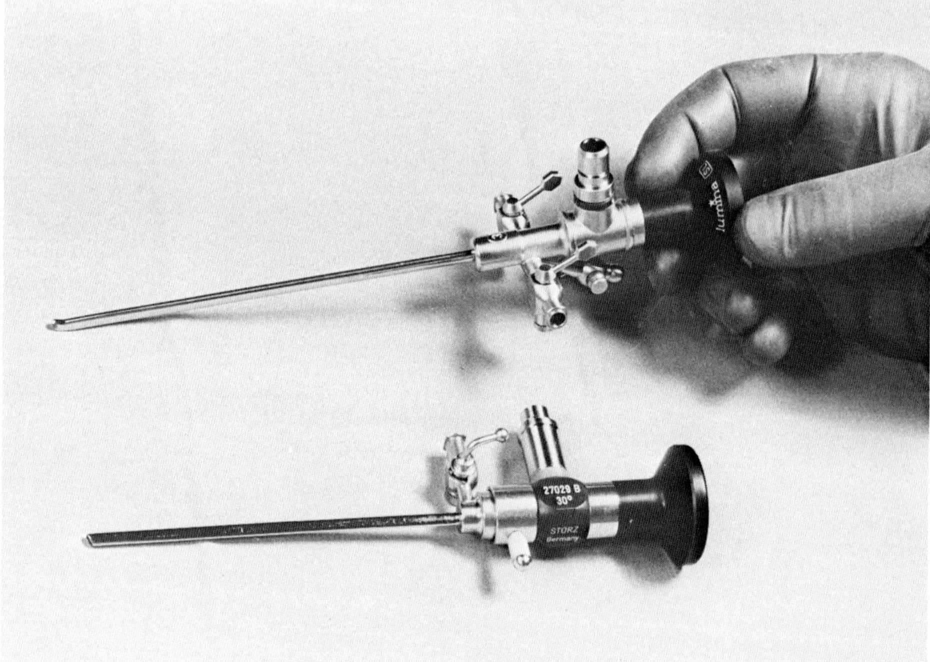

Figure 9-5. *Two of the modern pediatric endoscopes available for use in small infants. Both are 8 F caliber. Above is the model available from Richard Wolf Inc. It has two irrigating ports and a catheterizing channel that will accept a 3 F ureteral catheter for retrograde study or to fulgurate urethral valves. The telescope and sheath are a single assembly. Below is model available from Karl Storz. It lacks a catheterizing channel, but with more light bundles, it gives much better visualization of the anatomy. When an especially small male infant is examined, the telescope can be removed from the sheath and introduced by itself, after first filling the bladder with irrigating solution. In resection of valves in the newborn we first visualize the anatomy with the Storz instrument. Once all anatomic landmarks are seen the Wolf instrument is used to fulgurate the valves. Having both of these fine instruments available has avoided need for perineal urethrostomy in recent years, even in the neonate.*

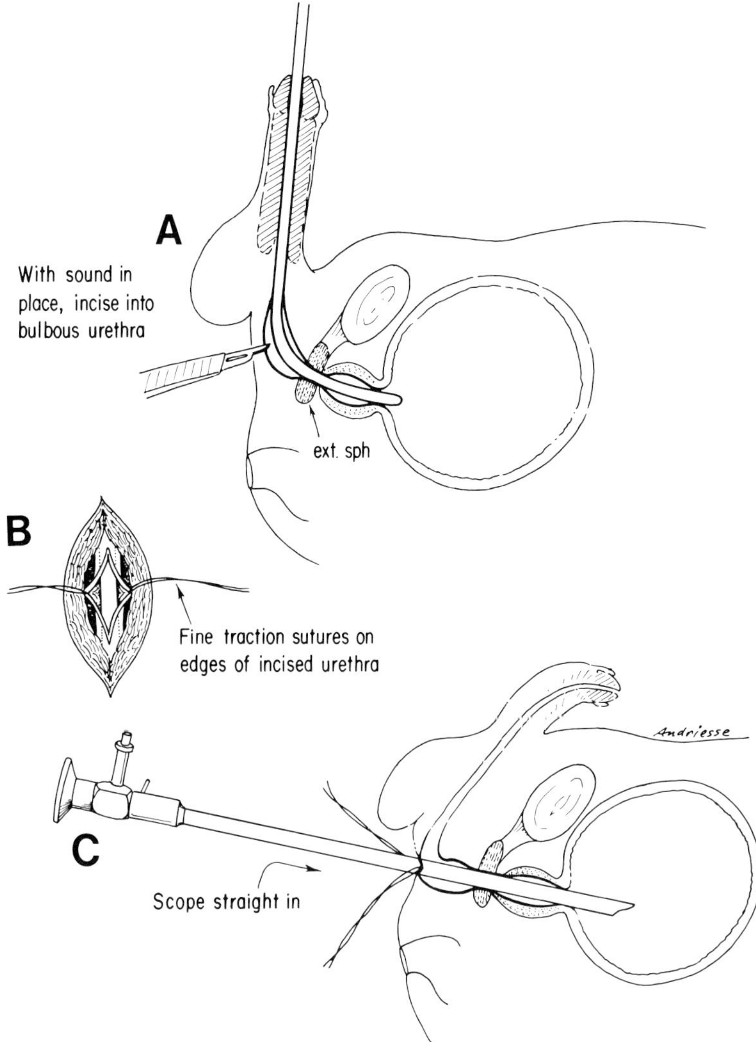

Figure 9-6. *Technique for perineal urethrostomy. (A) With patient in lithotomy position a sound is passed into urethra. An incision is made through perineum onto the sound in the bulbous urethra. (B) Fine traction sutures are placed on edges of urethra. (C) An endoscope can be passed through the perineal urethrostomy to visualize the bladder or fulgurate valves. The site of a perineal urethrostomy done in this manner is generally just distal to the external urethral sphincter. Complications we have observed from this procedure include stricture of the urethra and injury to the external urethral sphincter at 6 o'clock.*

Urologic telescopes are available with viewing angles that vary from 0° (straight ahead viewing) to 90° (right-angle viewing). In most cases we prefer to use the 30° foroblique lens. This is satisfactory for inspecting the urethra and also the entire bladder. Starting at a particular reference point, such as the air bubble in the dome of the bladder or the interureteric ridge, the telescope can be alternately advanced and pulled back, inspecting one quadrant of the bladder from cephalad to caudad, then repeating this maneuver while rotating the scope through 360°. This permits visualization of every aspect of the bladder. We use the 0° lens principally in the pediatric resectoscope, where that angle is necessary to visualize the cutting loop. The 0° lens may also be required to pass through strictures where a straight-ahead view is best.

Irrigating Solution

Water is used for most endoscopy procedures. It gives superior clarity of vision compared to electrolyte solutions, which give a hazy view because solute diffuses light. The solution should be warmed to body temperature. A prolonged endoscopic procedure in a small baby can cause precipitous cooling if the solution is at room temperature. A heating blanket beneath the child is another safeguard against hypothermia. In special circumstances, such as cases where the bladder has been augmented by bowel mucosa that can rapidly absorb the irrigating solution, it is better to use an electrolyte-containing solution to avert possible water intoxication. We prefer to attach a length of ordinary suction tubing to one of the irrigating ports on the panendoscope, alternating filling through the water intake and opening the drainage tube to evacuate water from the bladder. With the end of the tube placed in a bucket on the floor, there is a siphon effect to increase the speed of emptying. This provides constant washing away of blood around the lens system or bubbles during a procedure that involves electrofulguration. It also keeps the operator's lap dry! For children I prefer this technique as compared with using a special endoscopy table with a pull-out water-collecting unit, which is indeed useful in adult cases such as prostatic resection.

Identification of Ureteral Orifices

For the beginner, rapid identification of the ureteral orifices is the first milestone. This can be soon mastered by viewing the bladder neck posterior at 6 o'clock, advancing the telescope until the interureteric ridge comes into view, and then rotating the telescope to the right or left along the interureteric ridge until the orifice is encountered. In some bladders the orifices may be hard to identify, such as cases with severe cystitis, heavy trabeculation, or multiple cellules. Intravenous indigo carmine, together with a fluid load, can aid in their identification. If the patient is not dehydrated, blue will squirt from the ureteral orifices in a few minutes. This is *not* a reliable help in identification of an ectopic ureteral orifice outside of the bladder; an ectopic orifice is usually associated with a dysplastic segment of kidney that concentrates poorly. A segment poorly seen by intravenous pyelography will not excrete the blue dye in good concentration.

Learning to recognize normal anatomy is important so that the surgeon will recognize those findings that are slightly abnormal as well as those that are obviously pathologic. For example, the normal ureteral orifice is elliptically shaped, is at the end of a well-defined interureteric ridge, and is located in the bladder trigone (Figure 9-7). It has a submucosal tunnel 5–10 mm long which prevents reflux. In the male the tunnel can be demonstrated by passing a calibrated ureteral catheter into it. In females this can be demonstrated also by passing a malleable probe through the urethra, alongside the panendoscope, inserting it into the orifice, and elevating the submucosal segment of ureter (Figure 9-7). Configuration and location of orifices can prove important in assessing the indications for correcting vesicoureteral reflux. For example, if reflux is not great in amount, the upper tracts are normal, and the

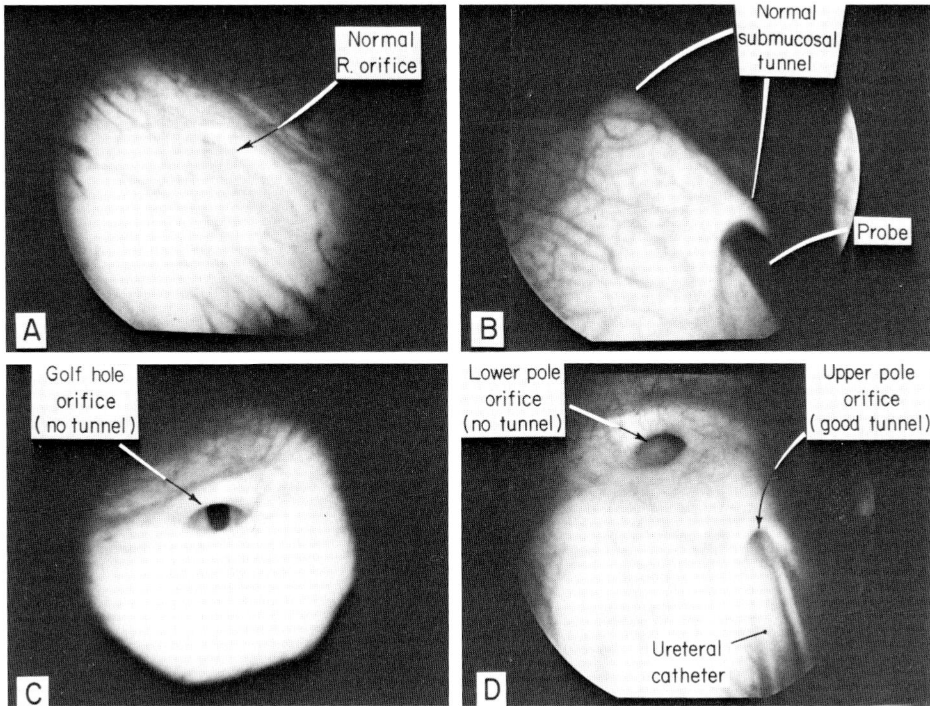

Figure 9-7. *Endoscopic appearance of urethral orifices. (A) Normal right orifice with elliptical shape, delicate mucosal edges, and good muscle backing. (B) Malleable probe introduced through urethra (female) next to endoscope, elevating anterior wall of distal ureter. The submucosal tunnel is 10 mm long, which provides a valvelike mechanism to prevent reflux. (C) Golf hole ureter in patient with massive reflux. There is no submucosal segment of ureter. It is possible to look several centimeters directly up this ureter. In some, dilatation is great enough that the panendoscope can be passed its full length directly up the ureter. (D) Typical anatomy of duplex collecting system with selective reflux to lower pole. Note that upper orifice, which drains lower pole, has golf hole configuration and no tunnel. The lower orifice, which drains upper pole, has normal configuration, a good submucosal tunnel, and no reflux.*

anatomy is close to normal, there is a good likelihood that this reflux will disappear in time. Nonoperative treatment is indicated. On the other hand, if the ureteral orifice has the appearance of a golf hole or gopher hole, is laterally located, and lacks a submucosal tunnel, reflux is unlikely to disappear. Operative correction is preferred. Duplicated collecting system is commonly associated with reflux. Most often the lower hole, which drains the upper pole, has a good submucosal segment and no reflux. Conversely, the upper hole, which drains the lower pole of the kidney, may lack a submucosal tunnel and allow selective reflux to the lower pole of the kidney (Figure 9-7). Occasionally there is reflux into both segments, which lie side by side instead of one above the other, so that both lack a tunnel. Also in a few cases the upper pole will demonstrate reflux but not the lower pole. Invariably the upper pole orifice is too caudad, located in the bladder neck or urethra, where it has no submucosal tunnel.

Cystoscopy should always include careful inspection of the urethra. It can be the site of much abnormality that can be overlooked on radiographic examination (Figures 9-8, 9-9, 9-10).

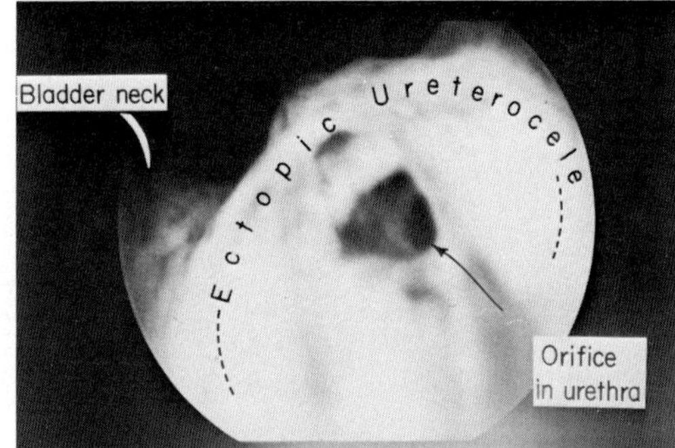

Figure 9-8. *Endoscopic appearance of ectopic ureterocele emptying into proximal urethra just distal to the bladder neck in 1-year-old girl. Note flaring orifice of ureterocele from water stream of panendoscope.*

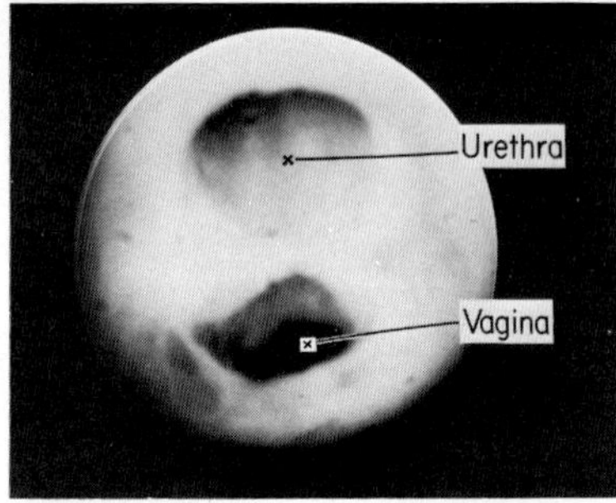

Figure 9-9. *Ectopic opening of vagina into urethra, at lower edge of external urethral sphincter, in patient with mixed gonadal dysgenesis.*

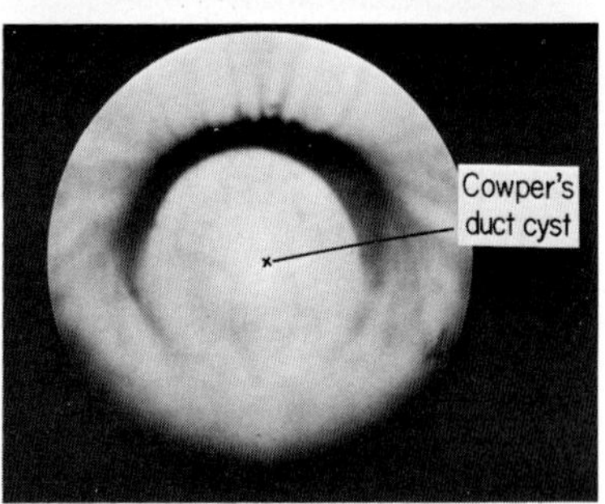

Figure 9-10. *Cowper's duct cyst on floor of bulbous urethra of 8-year-old boy.*

Retrograde Catheterization of Ureters

The standard woven ureteral catheters used in adult urology are too stiff for use in small infants. We prefer using special soft clear plastic catheters furnished in sizes 3 and 4 F*. Initial placement in the ureteral orifice is facilitated by a wire stylet with which the catheters are furnished. As the catheter is advanced up the ureter, the stylet is pulled back gradually.

The need for retrograde pyelography has diminished greatly in my practice since we began using antegrade pyelography (Figures 9-11, 9-12). In cases of hydronephrosis we much prefer antegrade pyelography to the old-fashioned retrograde studies. A No. 22 spinal needle is passed below the 12th rib into the dilated collecting system. Contrast medium is infused while observing fluoroscopically. This

*Available from Cunningham Woodland Inc., Boston, Massachusetts 02190.

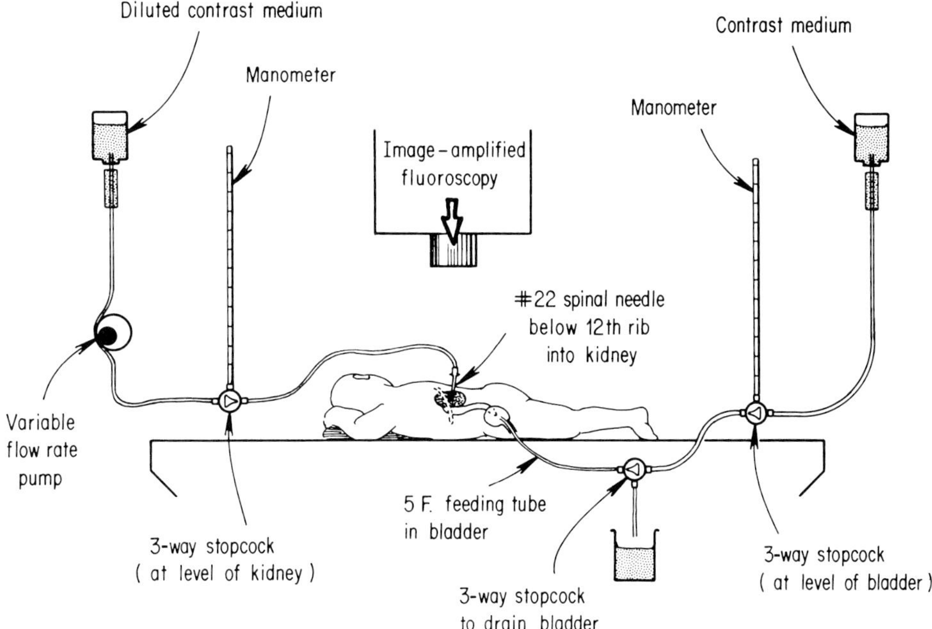

Figure 9-11. *Schematic diagram of antegrade pyelography with pressure–perfusion study. Antegrade pyelography in the conscious patient has supplanted retrograde pyelogram examination under anesthesia in many of our patients with hydronephrosis caused by various obstructions in the urinary tract. In addition to excellent delineation of anatomy, it makes possible fluoroscopy with image amplification and pressure measurements to determine gradients at the site of obstruction. (From Hendren WH: Megaureter, in J. Hartwell Harrison, et al: Campell's Urology (ed 4). Philadelphia, W.B. Saunders, 1979. With permission.)*

outlines anatomy without artifact from a retrograde catheter. The procedure is performed under fluoroscopic control. The patient is examined awake, in prone position. Sedation may be used in infants or young children. Today we use retrograde examination only when antegrade study is not feasible. Antegrade studies also allow pressure–perfusion determination, i.e., the Whittaker test,[3] to measure the degree of possible obstruction. If retrograde examination is to be performed in a nondilated system, only a small amount of contrast should be injected (1–2 ml in a baby, 3–5 ml in a larger patient). In a dilated system, however, one can aspirate a known amount and replace it with the same volume of contrast medium. These precautions guard against overfilling the kidney, causing pyelotubular backflow and absorption of the contrast medium into the blood stream.

Passing a retrograde catheter, even a small and soft one, past an obstructive lesion such as obstructive megaureter or ureteropelvic junction obstruction, can cause edema and total obstruction in a few hours. Another hazard is introduction of bacteria, which can cause pyonephrosis in a kidney which is draining poorly. Therefore, it is best to delay retrograde ureteral catheterization in such cases until the time of the actual operative procedure, just before obstruction is to be relieved.

Retrograde study is a useful way to visualize the upper tracts in patients with allergy to intravenous administration of the agent. Most commonly this is encountered in patients who have undergone previous urologic surgery, who after repeated

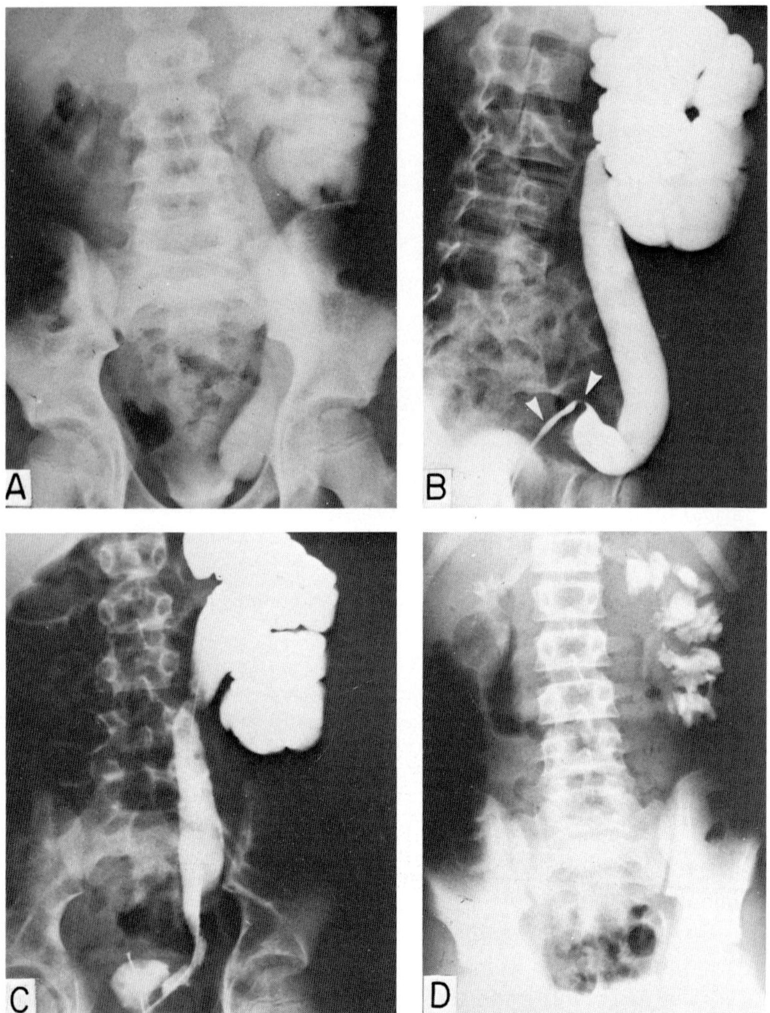

Figure 9-12. *Typical case with hydronephrosis demonstrating value of antegrade pyelography. (A) IVP showing left hydroureteronephrosis and normal right side. Cystogram was normal. (B) Antegrade pyelogram showing very long narrow distal segment of ureter (arrows). This segment was resected and lower part of dilated ureter was tapered and reimplanted into the bladder. (C) Injection of ureteral catheter stent 12 days after lower ureter repair. Note that length of lower ureter tapered extends to level of iliac vessels, not higher. (D) IVP 6 months later showing marked improvement. (Reproduced with permission from Hendren WH: Reconstructive surgery of the urinary tract in children, in Ravitch MM, et al (eds): Current Problems in Surgery. Copyright © 1977 by Year Book Medical Publishers, Inc., Chicago.)*

examinations have become sensitized to the contrast medium. Subsequent intravenous administration of the agent may be dangerous. Retrograde injection is a suitable alternative. Alternatively, radionuclide scanning can be used, but this does not give the anatomic detail needed in some cases.

Ureteroceles can pose a special problem (see Figure 26, p. vi). In some the orifice to the ureterocele is too small to admit even a small catheter. We have found the following technique useful. The tip of a 22-gauge needle is cut across with heavy scissors and is inserted into the end of a 3 F ureteral catheter. Another 22 needle is inserted into the other end of the ureteral catheter. With the wire stylet in the ureteral catheter, this needle-catheter can puncture the ureterocele endoscopically. Contrast medium is injected after removing the stylet. This needle-catheter can be made in a few minutes. An alternative technique is puncture of the ureterocele using a spinal needle passed into the bladder suprapubically while viewing endoscopically.

In recent years cross-trigone ureteral reimplantation, introduced by Cohen[4] has gained wide usage. It can be difficult to retrograde a cross-trigone reimplant. We have had better success in these cases by emptying most of the water from the bladder to collapse the intramural ureter. This facilitates passing the catheter. Another trick is to bend the stylet to an angle to get the catheter started, extracting the wire as the catheter is advanced. Sometimes it proves impossible to retrograde this type of reimplant from below. An alternative is to pass a needle into the bladder percutaneously, and pass through it the retrograde catheter into the ureter while viewing from below. Endoscopy lends itself well to acquiring useful little tricks after long practice.

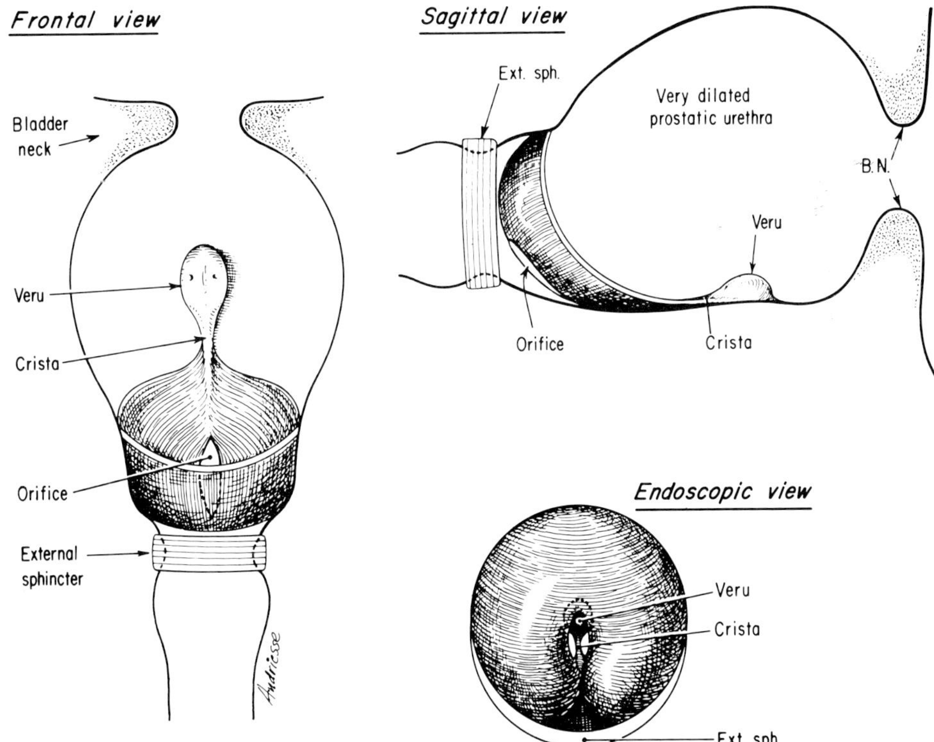

Figure 9-13. *The most common anatomic configuration in males with severe urethral valves obstructing prostatic urethra. Note valve leaflets arising from crista urethralis, just distal to verumontanum, and fusing dorsally to form a diaphragmlike obstruction. When viewed from below there is often a narrow slitlike opening between the leaflets, usually at 6 o'clock. Valves are best viewed with the bladder full and the prostatic urethra distended. The 12 o'clock confluence of valve leaflets is often adjacent to the external urethral sphincter. Pulling a hook or cutting loop toward the operator in cutting the valve at 12 o'clock can sever the external urethral sphincter, which may cause postoperative incontinence.*

Urethral Valves

Urethral valves are much more common than generally appreciated.[5] As with all pathologic conditions, they occur in a spectrum from mild to severe. At the mild end of the spectrum is an older boy with voiding symptoms including bed wetting, day wetting, urgency, frequency, and sometimes a poor stream. At the severe end of the spectrum is the young infant with marked hydronephrosis and sometimes a weak, dribbling stream. Some surgeons have advocated using the pediatric resectoscope for destroying valves, but I prefer using a wire electrode through a straight endoscope sheath. A resectoscope sheath is too large in small babies; it cannot be passed in an infant male except through a perineal urethrostomy. Even in older boys it may be too tight, leading to urethral injury. Furthermore, a resectoscope loop is relatively large in surface area and gives less precise destruction of valve leaflets than a wire electrode. A Bugbee electrode can be used, but in most cases we use the wire stylet of a 3 F woven ureteral catheter as the electrode and the catheter as the insulating sheath (see p. 63). To the proximal end of the stylet is attached the Bovie unit. A short segment of wire is advanced beyond the end of the sheath to serve as the cutting electrode. The anatomy of severe urethral valves is shown in Figures 9-13, 9-14, and 9-15. The technique for their destruction is shown in Figures 9-16 and 9-17. Cutting current is used in brief bursts. Usually we commence with a cut in the 12 o'clock position to incise the dorsal confluence of valve leaflets that forms the obstructive diaphragm. In some cases this is all that is needed. In the majority, however, there remains the base of the valve leaflets on each side. The left leaflet is incised at 5 o'clock and the right leaflet at 7 o'clock. This creates a cloverleaf defect. This is a much safer and more precise technique for destroying valves than using a resectoscope loop. Pulling a resectoscope loop toward oneself in resecting valves risks injury to the external urethral sphincter, especially at 12 o'clock, where the external sphincter is very near.

The diagnosis of valves can nearly always be made from the voiding cystourethrogram. Endoscopic resection of the valves in a newborn in my opinion poses one of the greatest challenges in pediatric urologic endoscopy. Years ago they were resected by splitting the public symphysis and excising them under direct vision. Today we visualize them using the Storz 8 F infant panendoscope (see Figure 28, p. vi). This delicate instrument gives superb visualization. However, it lacks a catheterizing channel. After the anatomy is viewed with this instrument, the Wolf 8 F infant panendoscope is used to do the resection. It has a catheterizing channel that will accept the 3 F catheter with its wire stylet. It has less brilliant illumination, but this is not so important once the anatomy has been clearly visualized through the Storz instrument. We have found this combination of instruments to be ideal in actual practice. Certainly both of these firms manufacture instruments of superb quality, as do several other companies in this field. A larger sheath can be used in older boys, giving the advantage of faster water flow.

Rarely there is an indication to widen the bladder neck endoscopically. It is not necessary to do this with the resectoscope loop. When brief bursts of cutting current are used, an electrode will divide the hypertrophied muscle and widen the neck just as effectively as if it were actually resected. We have seen virtually no indication in childhood for circumferential resection of the bladder neck, which is likely to cause irreparable scarring. In our experience most clinicians accurately diagnose cases of severe urethral valves, which would be expected since they are

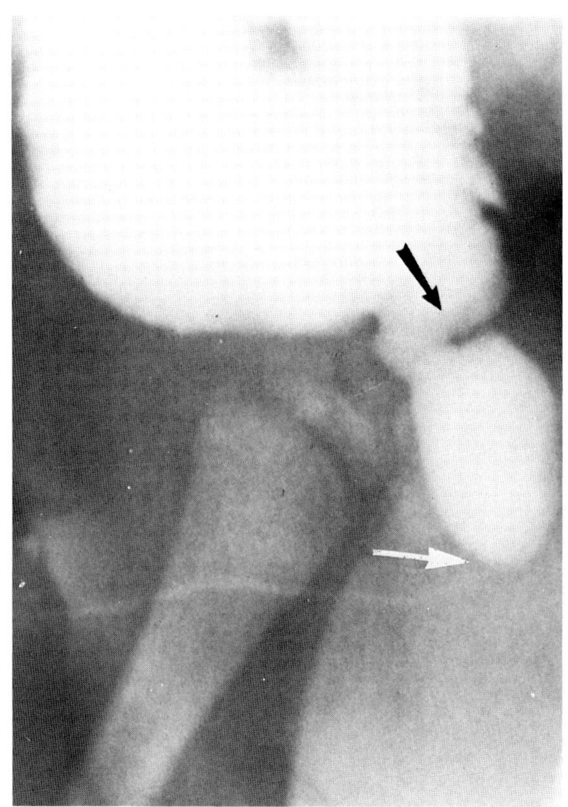

Figure 9-14. *Voiding cystourethrogram in newborn male with severe urethral obstruction from type I valves (white arrow). Note threadlike stream in penile urethra and severe dilatation of prostatic urethra. There is secondary hypertrophy of bladder neck (black arrow) and massive reflux up both dilated ureters.*

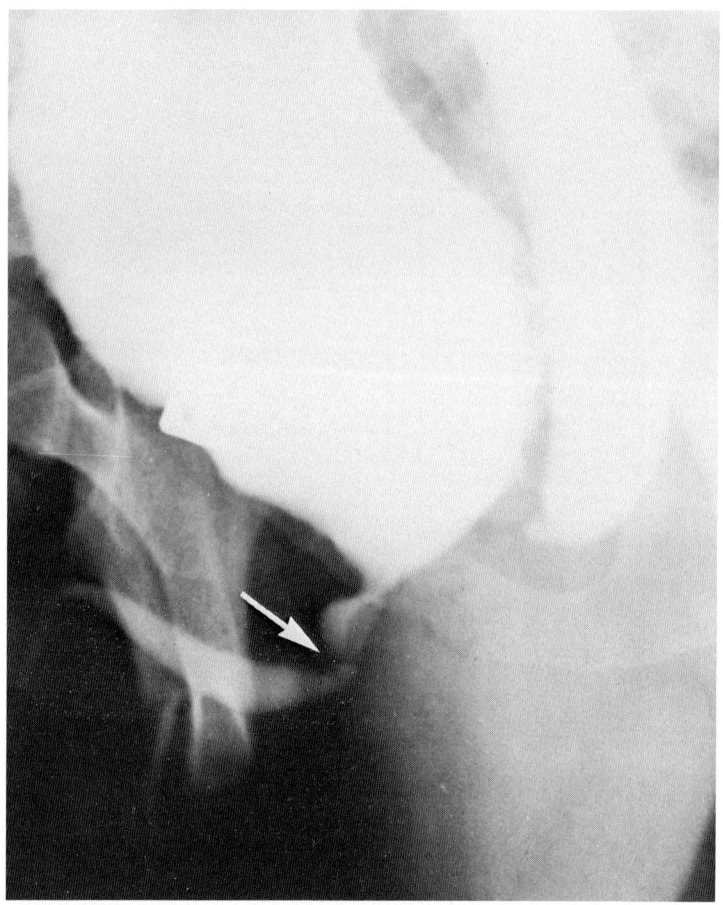

Figure 9-15. *Severe urethral valves (arrow) in a 6-year-old boy referred to endocrinology service for "diabetes insipidus." The history included urinary frequency, day and night wetting, and polyuria. Note markedly different appearance of prostatic urethra in this case compared with that in Figure 9-14. Both had severe type I urethral valves. In some cases the crista is very elongated, and the prostatic urethra is very dilated. In others, like this case, it is not. This patient had severe bilateral hydronephrosis. Note massive reflux up dilated ureter. Blood chemical values showed elevated blood urea nitrogen of 40 mg/100 ml, and creatinine clearance was reduced to 50 percent of normal (see Figure 9-17 for photographs of valves in this patient).*

SEVERE TYPE I VALVES

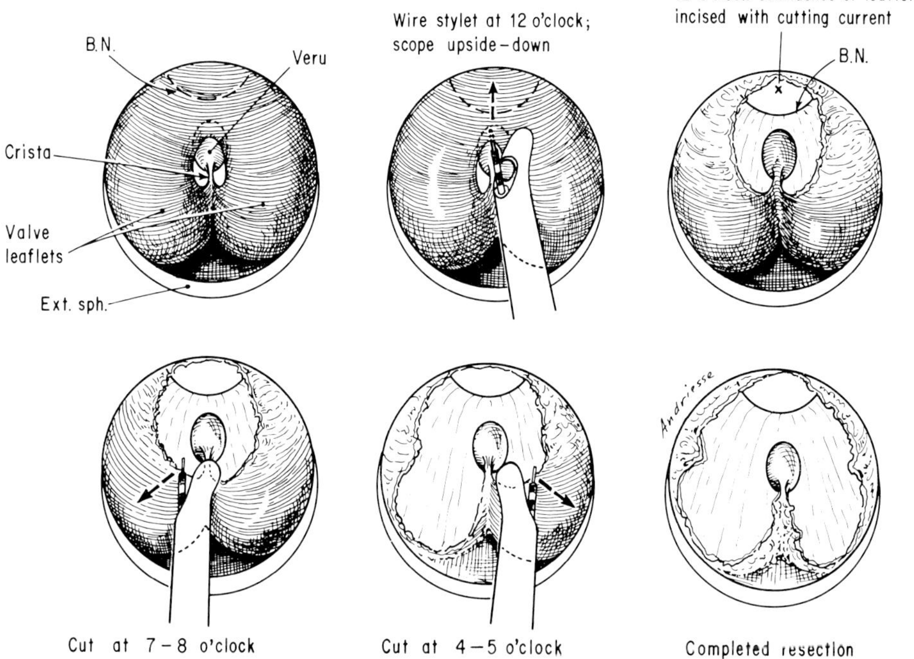

Figure 9-16. *Technique for resecting severe type I valves. The valves are visualized with the bladder full and the irrigating reservoir at least 3 feet above the patient to distend the prostatic urethra. A 3 F ureteral catheter and its wire stylet are used as a cutting electrode, attaching a Bovie unit to the distal end of the wire and advancing a few millimeters of wire beyond the cut end of the catheter to act as a cutting electrode. When this electrode is advanced into the field of vision it is best to have the endoscope in the bladder to avoid inadvertently puncturing the side wall of the urethra. Then, with the electrode clearly in view of the foroblique lens, the scope is withdrawn until the valve is reached. It is then turned 180°, to start with a 12 o'clock cut. Very brief applications of cutting current are used to incise the dorsal confluence of the valve leaflets to their point of attachment on the roof of the prostatic urethra. It is important not to cut distal to that point, where the external voluntary urethral sphincter is located. In some cases this 12 o'clock cut is all that is needed to completely relieve the obstruction. In others there remains a sail-like fold on each side, attached to the crista urethralis. The right one can be cut at 7–8 o'clock and the left one at 4–5 o'clock. This technique, using a fine wire or fine Bugbee electrode, is very precise and is possible without touching the verumontanum, the side wall of the urethra, or the external sphincter. The urethral valves should not be fulgurated in a defunctioned urethra, for that can cause stricture if the patient is not intermittently voiding through the area.*

usually quite obvious both radiographically and endoscopically. On the other hand, less severe cases of valves are often not diagnosed, although they are quite common in clinical practice. It stands to reason that mild cases should occur, since all developmental malformations do in fact occur in a spectrum which ranges from mild to severe. A mild case is shown in Figure 9-18, whose presenting symptoms were frequency, urgency, and day and night wetting. In milder cases the 12 o'clock confluence of valves may be less striking or even absent. Endoscopic resection in that case may require only the lateral cuts. A motion picture showing the spectrum

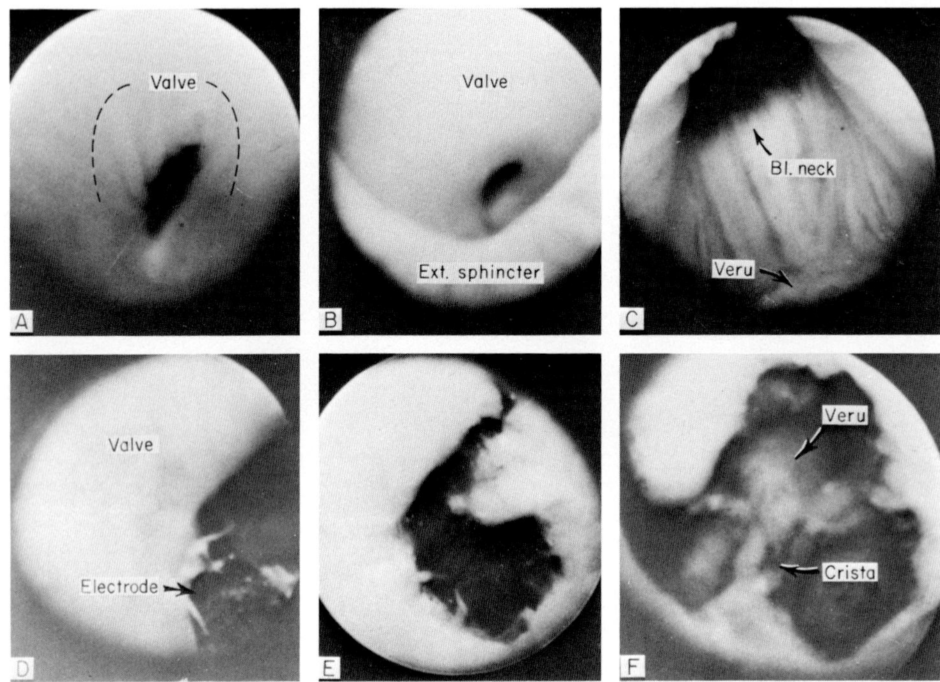

Figure 9-17. *Valves of patient shown in Figure 9-15. (A) Closeup view of valves, which form a diaphragm. (B) Scope is pulled slightly more distally to show the position of external sphincter with relation to valves. The 12 o'clock component of the valves inserts very close to the external sphincter, whereas the origin of the valves from the crista urethralis is at a distance from the sphincter at 6 o'clock. (C) Moderately hypertrophied bladder neck, which should be left alone initially. (D) Electrode about to cut left valve leaflet. (E) After completing 12 o'clock cut and 4–5 o'clock cut on left side. Right lateral leaflet still visible. (F) After incising right leaflet. Note cloverleaf opening where valves were. Clear view of verumontanum. External urethral sphincter still intact, but not shown in this illustration. (Reproduced with permission from Hendren WH: Reconstructive surgery of the urinary tract in children, in Ravitch MM, et al (eds): Current Problems in Surgery. Copyright © 1977 by Year Book Medical Publishers, Inc., Chicago.)*

of valves and their destruction is available from the film libraries of the American College of Surgeons, Norwich Eaton Laboratories, and Karl Storz Endoscopy–America.[6]

Urethral Stricture

Urethral strictures are sometimes encountered in children. Some are congenital. Others result from unskilled endoscopy causing trauma. Some are caused by external trauma, such as the straddle injury on a bicycle. Passing an endoscope in a case of stricture must always be done under direct vision. Blind insertion of an instrument can create a false passage. A fine ureteral catheter should be passed through the stricture into the bladder, followed by a small endoscope. If the stricture is too small or irregular, a pigtail filiform may be useful to get through it, after which followers of increasing size can be passed to open the stricture enough to accept a panendoscope. After visualization, decision can be made as to how it should best be treated. Some can be treated as a valve by incising with a cutting electrode.

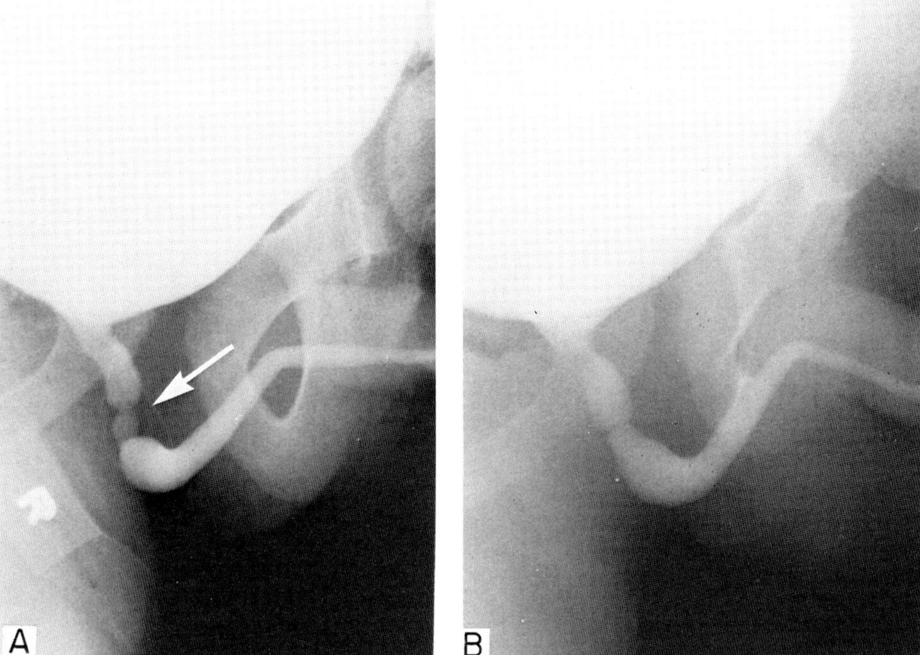

Figure 9-18. *Mild urethral valves in a 12-year-old boy whose urinary tract was investigated after one episode of infection. An older brother had severe urethral valves operated on previously. Urodynamic study showed low flow rate with flat curve and slightly elevated voiding pressure. (A) Preoperative voiding cystourethrogram. Note slight indentation of urethra just distal to verumontanum (arrow), 1 cm above external urethral sphincter. (B) Postoperative study 2 years later. Voiding pressures were normal and flow two times greater.*

Others are best treated by excision and reanastomosis of the urethra or by patch graft using penile skin or bladder mucosa. Some can be treated by incision with the cold knife blade attached to a pediatric resectoscope and an inlying nonreactive catheter for 2–3 weeks. Open resection is needed in some cases.

Nephroscopy

It is sometimes necessary to look directly into the kidney. Most commonly this is done during stone surgery. Although flexible nephroscopes are available, they currently leave much to be desired in clarity of vision. The rigid nephroscope (also used for choledochoscopy) made by Storz has great optical clarity but has the disadvantage of a fixed right-angle configuration. By mobilizing the kidney and inserting the right-angle instrument through a pyelotomy incision, good visualization is achieved in larger patients. The interior of the kidney can also be inspected by using a straight panendoscope through a nephrotomy in a dilated calyx. We have used nephroscopy in a few postoperative pyeloplasty cases where drainage was partly blocked. If a nephrostomy tube is in place and the tract is well established, a straight panendoscope can be inserted gently directly into the kidney, visualizing the recent ureteropelvic junction anastomosis. In two cases edematous mucosa was seen to be the problem. In another an actual stricture was observed.

Conclusion

Pediatric urologic endoscopy is an important component of the surgery for genitourinary problems in infants and children. It is essential to have suitably miniaturized equipment to perform these procedures safely. As in most types of surgery, practice of this discipline confers increasing expertise.

References

1. Gans SL, Berci G: Advances in endoscopy of infants and children. J Pediatr Surg 6:199–233, 1971
2. Hendren WH, Crawford JD: Adrenogenital syndrome: the anatomy of the anomaly and its repair. J Pediatr Surg 4:49, 1969
3. Whittaker RH: Methods of assessing obstruction in dilated ureters. Br J Urol 45:15, 1973
4. Cohen SJ: Ureterozystoneostomie: Eine neue antireflux Technik, Aktuel. Urol 6:1, 1975
5. Hendren WH: Posterior urethral valves in boys: a broad clinical spectrum. J Urol 106:298, 1971
6. Hendren WH: Urethral Valves: Diagnosis and Endoscopic Resection, motion picture. Film no. 984, film libraries of American College of Surgeons; Film no. 850, Eaton Laboratories, Norwich, also available from Storz Endoscopy–America.

Thoracoscopy

CHAPTER 10

Bradley M. Rodgers

The technique of thoracoscopy was first described by Jacobaeus, in 1910.[1] Using cystoscopic instruments, crude by modern standards, Jacobaeus was able to view the pleural space and successfully dissect fibrinous pleural adhesions. With few refinements, the technique enjoyed wide popularity in the early portion of this century, primarily for the lysis of pleural adhesions prior to instituting pneumothorax therapy for pulmonary tuberculosis. With the advent of modern thoracic surgery and better anesthetic techniques, however, thoracoscopy fell into relative disuse. As superior optical instruments have been developed for use in bronchoscopy, several individuals have re-examined the technique of thoracoscopy and have applied it for thoracic diagnosis.[2-4] In July 1975 we began to utilize the technique of thoracoscopy for thoracic diagnosis in children. Initially, our primary indication for thoracoscopy was for the diagnosis of diffuse pulmonary infiltrates in immunosuppressed children, but with increasing experience we have expanded our indications for its use.

Methods and Results

Between July 1, 1975 and January 1, 1980 we performed 86 thoracoscopy procedures in 80 patients 20 years of age or younger. Six patients were thoracoscoped on two occasions and one individual underwent four separate thoracoscopy procedures for intrathoracic diagnosis. The instruments employed in this procedure are manufactured by Karl Storz* and are primarily designed for laparoscopy in children (Figure 10-1). The telescopes employ the Hopkins rod lens system, and both the biopsy forceps and suction equipment are insulated to allow electrocoagulation. For infants and children under the age of 2 years, the 3.75-mm O.D. infant trocar (26180) is used in conjunction with the small, straight viewing telescope (27018A). The 5-mm O.D. pediatric trocar (26172C) is used in larger patients. This trocar allows passage of a larger, straight viewing telescope (27015A) and biopsy forceps (26175DB).

All of these procedures have been performed in the general operating suite. The patients fast for 6 hours prior to the procedure and usually receive premedication consisting of atropine (0.2 mg/kg body weight), pentobarbitol sodium (4 mg/kg) and meperidine hydrochloride (1 mg/kg). The manner of intraoperative anesthetic

*Karl Storz KG, Tuttlingen, West Germany; Storz Endoscopy–America, Culver City, California.

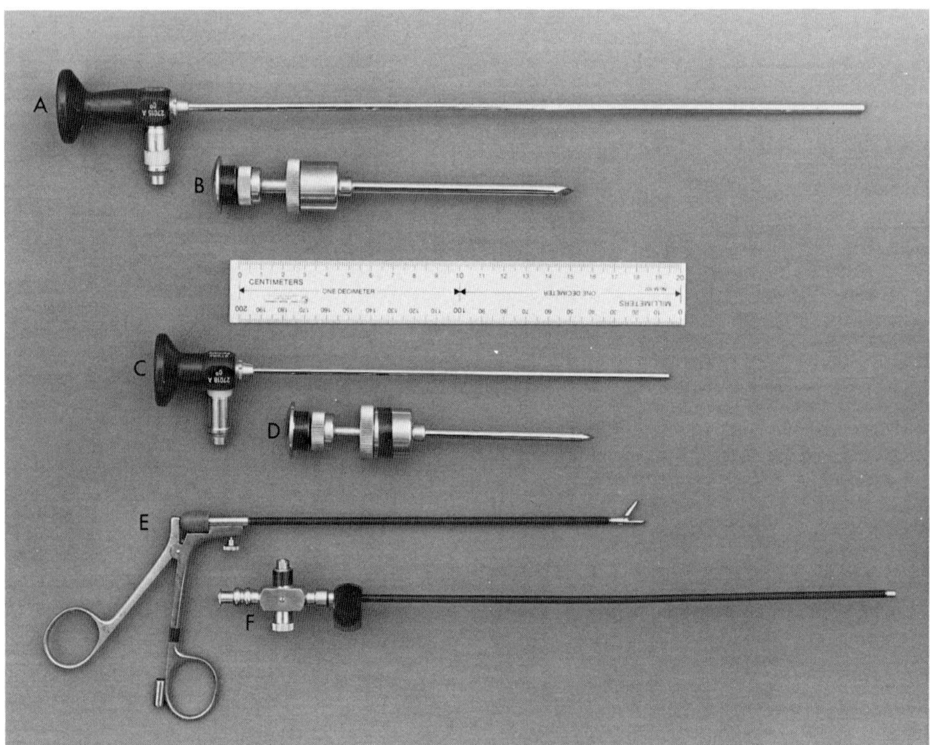

Figure 10-1. *Thoracoscopy instruments. (A) Large, straight viewing Hopkins rod lens telescope. (B) Pediatric thoracoscopy trocar with stylet inserted. (C) Small, straight viewing Hopkins rod lens telescope. (D) Infant thoracoscopy trocar with stylet inserted. (E) Insulated biopsy forceps that passes through the infant thoracoscopy trocar. (F) Insulated suction cannula that passes through the infant thoracoscopy trocar. (From Rodgers BM, Moazam F, Talbert JL: Thoracoscopy: early diagnosis of interstitial pneumonitis in the immunologically suppressed child. Chest 75: 126–130, 1979. With permission.)*

management has been modified as we have gained experience with this technique. In small infants and children under the age of 2 years, general anesthesia with endotracheal intubation is currently employed. With this technique, it is important that the patient be breathing spontaneously during the performance of thoracoscopy. With the use of positive pressure endotracheal ventilation, it is very difficult to achieve a sufficient pneumothorax to allow a satisfactory view within the chest. For older patients, a combination of unilateral stellate ganglion block and intercostal nerve block with Marcaine* anesthesia has proven most satisfactory. Use of regional anesthesia has markedly reduced the necessity for intravenous anesthetic agents. The stellate ganglion block reduces the cough reflex initiated by traction on the visceral pleural surface with the thoracoscopy instruments. The intercostal nerve block completely eliminates the pain from the parietal pleura in the region of insertion of the thoracoscopy trocars. Intravenous anesthetics, such as Ketaject,† are used as necessary to achieve very light sedation during the procedure.

After suitable anesthesia has been achieved in these patients, they are situated on the operating table in an appropriate position, depending upon the region of the pathologic condition within the hemithorax. The patients are allowed to spontaneously breathe a high concentration of oxygen by placing a face mask close to their mouth and nose. After prepping and draping the chest the thoracoscopy trocar is inserted through an appropriate intercostal space and a pneumothorax is induced. When the stylet is removed from the trocar, air is trapped within the hemithorax by the valve within the trocar, thereby allowing complete visualization of the intrathoracic structures. A second trocar is inserted next to the first for insertion of the biopsy and suction instruments. Biopsy specimens of the pulmonary parenchyma are obtained by shearing the pulmonary tissue free as the forceps are withdrawn into the trocar. Electrocoagulation is used only after the biopsy specimen has been obtained and then only if there is significant bleeding from the pulmonary surface. Following the completion of the procedure the trocars are removed and an intercostal chest catheter is inserted and left to suction for at least 12 hours.

For the purposes of review, the indications for thoracoscopy have been divided into four major categories: pulmonary parenchymal biopsy in immunosuppressed patients; pulmonary parenchymal biopsy in nonimmunosuppressed patients; biopsy of intrathoracic tumors; and miscellaneous therapeutic indications (Table 10-1).

*Marcaine (bupivacaine hydrochloride), Breon Laboratories, Inc., 90 Park Avenue, New York, New York 10016.

† Ketaject (ketamine hydrochloride), Bristol Laboratories, Syracuse, New York 13201.

Table 10-1
Indications for Thoracoscopy in Children

Immunosuppressed	42
Pulmonary infiltrates	15
Tumors	24
Other	5
Total	86

Pulmonary Parenchymal Biopsy in Immunosuppressed Patients

The technique of thoracoscopy was originally employed in an attempt to provide a safe and rapid technique for pulmonary tissue diagnosis in patients suspected of having *Pneumocystis carinii* pneumonia. In our early experience with thoracoscopy, the majority of the patients subjected to this procedure were immunosuppressed patients with diffuse pulmonary infiltrates. To date a total of 42 procedures have been performed in 38 immunosuppressed children (Table 10-2). The underlying diagnoses requiring the use of immunosuppressive agents included leukemia (19 patients), solid tumors (15 patients), renal transplantation (3 patients), and collagen vascular disease (1 patient). The patients were selected for thoracoscopy primarily on the basis of clinical symptoms and, to a lesser extent, on radiographic findings. In all cases the patients were febrile and noted to have dyspnea and tachypnea, often with an unproductive cough. The arterial blood gas determinations frequently revealed significant degrees of hypoxemia and hypocarbia, especially in the patients subsequently proven to have *Pneumocystis carinii* pneumonia. Evaluation of the chest roentgenograms proved to be of benefit in indicating a need for tissue diagnosis but was of less help in identifying those patients with actual *Pneumocystis carinii* pneumonia. The pulmonary roentgenographic findings in the patients with pneumocystis pneumonia varied from no abnormality to the presence of extensive bilateral interstitial pneumonia (Figure 10-2A,B). Since many of these patients had diffuse roentgenographic changes at the time of thoracoscopy, several pulmonary biopsies were generally obtained from each lobe of the lung. The thoracoscopy procedure was performed on the side of the maximal radiographic involvement, or on the right side in cases of equal involvement. The specimens obtained were immediately presented to the pathology department for touch preparations and frozen section as well as permanent section. Separate specimens were submitted for bacterial and, in some cases, viral cultures.

Pathologic evaluation of the pulmonary tissue obtained in 23 (55 percent) of these procedures revealed organisms characteristic for *Pneumocystis carinii* pneumonia. In these patients therapy was immediately instituted with trimethoprim/sulfamethoxazole (20 mg and 100 mg/kg/day). The patients found to have *Pneumocystis carinii* pneumonia had an overall survival of 83 percent, reflecting the efficacy of early diagnosis and therapy in these critically ill children. Visual inspection of the lung in patients with *Pneumocystis carinii* pneumonia revealed a pale appearance with edema manifest by blunting of the edges of the lung at the fissures (see Figure 30, p. vi).

The remaining diagnoses obtained at thoracoscopy in these immunosuppressed patients included bacterial pneumonia (8 procedures), viral pneumonia (4 proce-

Table 10–2
Thoracoscopy in Immunosuppressed Children

Patients	38
Procedures	42
Ages	2–20 years
Accuracy	98%

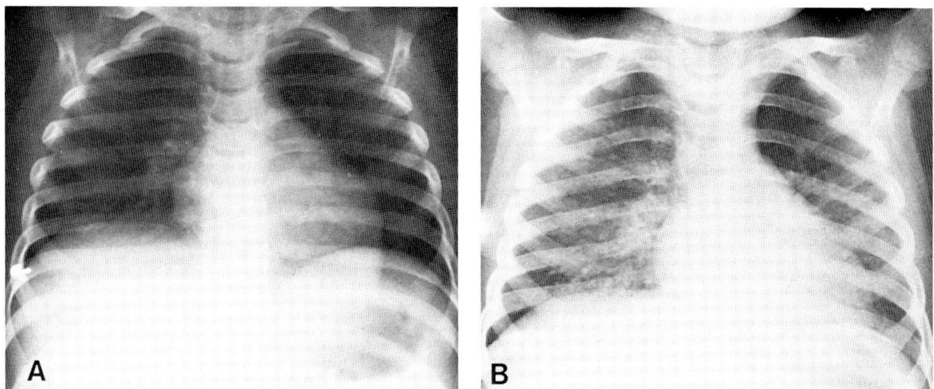

Figure 10-2. *(A) A 13-year-old boy receiving chemotherapy for acute leukemia had a 3-day history of fever and unproductive cough. Marked arterial hypoxemia was present while breathing room air. The frontal radiograph was interpreted as normal. Thoracoscopy with right lung biopsy revealed* Pneumocystis carinii *organisms. The patient was treated with trimethoprim/sulfamethoxazole for 4 months. Seven months later he returned with similar symptoms, and a frontal radiograph (B) revealed a characteristic picture of diffuse interstitial infiltrate with perihilar prominence. Left thoracoscopy and parenchymal biopsy revealed* Pneumocystis carinii *organisms and the patient was again placed on trimethoprim/sulfamethoxazole.*

dures), and interstitial fibrosis with alveolar hyperplasia, suggestive of irradiation or chemotherapy effects (7 procedures). The diagnostic accuracy of thoracoscopy in this group of patients has been 98 percent. In one 4-year-old child on chemotherapy for leukemia, thoracoscopy was performed for a pulmonary infiltrate (Figure 10-3). The tissue specimen revealed only interstitial fibrosis and alveolar hyperplasia. The persistence of roentgenographic findings and clinical symptoms prompted an open lung biopsy 2 weeks following thoracoscopy, and tissue obtained from this procedure revealed a leukemic infiltrate within the pulmonary parenchyma. In all other patients subjected to thoracoscopy, however, an accurate diagnosis has been obtained and response to therapy has been appropriate.

The complications noted following thoracoscopy in these critically ill children were more severe than those noted in any other group of patients in our series but,

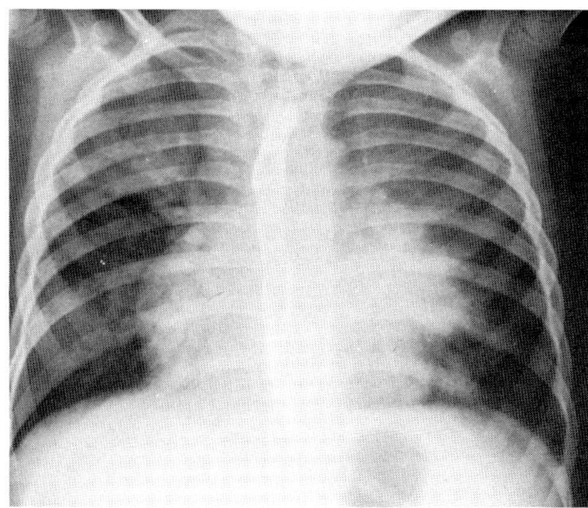

Figure 10-3. *Frontal chest radiograph of a 4-year-old child on chemotherapy for acute leukemia. Bilateral scattered pulmonary infiltrates were noted. Right thoracoscopy and pulmonary biopsy revealed interstitial fibrosis and alveolar hyperplasia. Open lung biopsy of the right upper lobe 2 weeks later revealed a leukemic infiltrate.*

nonetheless, were relatively mild. After four procedures a pneumothorax was noted, requiring either manipulation of the initial chest tube or insertion of a new chest tube for complete lung expansion. In none of these cases was a persistent bronchopleural fistula encountered. In each instance in which the complication of pneumothorax occurred, the pulmonary diagnosis was that of *Pneumocystis carinii* pneumonia. In these patients it has been noted on visual inspection at thoracoscopy that the pulmonary parenchyma is edematous and the lung compliance markedly reduced. These factors undoubtedly contribute to the high complication rate in these patients and have led us to recommend that the initial intercostal tube be left in place for 72 hours or longer following pulmonary biopsy in these patients. Two of these immunosuppressed children required transfusion following pulmonary biopsy. Both had severe thrombocytopenia and anemia prior to thoracoscopy. We have not hesitated to perform thoracoscopy and pulmonary biopsy in these immunosuppressed patients, despite the presence of profound thrombocytopenia in many of them. An accurate tissue diagnosis is of such importance to the appropriate management of these critically ill patients that the risk of postoperative bleeding following thoracoscopy appears more than justified. In both of the instances of bleeding, there was spontaneous resolution. Seven of these immunosuppressed patients died within 30 days of their thoracoscopy procedure. In none of these was it felt that the procedure itself contributed to their demise; rather, they succumbed to overwhelming pulmonary infection or neoplasm.

Pulmonary Parenchymal Biopsy in Nonimmunosuppressed Patients

Fifteen thoracoscopy procedures were performed in the same number of nonimmunosuppressed patients with undiagnosed pulmonary infiltrates (Table 10-3). The ages of these patients ranged between 2 months and 20 years. All of these patients had undergone the appropriate, less invasive, methods of pulmonary diagnosis or treatment prior to being presented for thoracoscopy. Six of the patients had undergone prior bronchoscopic evaluation without a specific diagnosis being achieved, and 3 had had nondiagnostic lung aspirates. The tissue diagnoses obtained by thoracoscopy in these patients included bacterial pneumonia (1 procedure), fungal pneumonia (3 procedures), tuberculosis (2 procedures), viral and mycoplasma pneumonia (2 procedures), and interstitial pneumonitis (3 procedures) (Figure 10-4). In each instance the pathologic area within the pulmonary parenchyma was easily identified at the time of thoracoscopy. These areas usually evidenced localized atelectatic or inflammatory changes, with a violaceous discoloration of the visceral pleural surface, or localized pleural adhesions. In these patients it has been

Table 10-3
Thoracoscopy in Children with Pulmonary Infiltrates

Patients	15
Procedures	15
Ages	2 months–20 years
Accuracy	93%

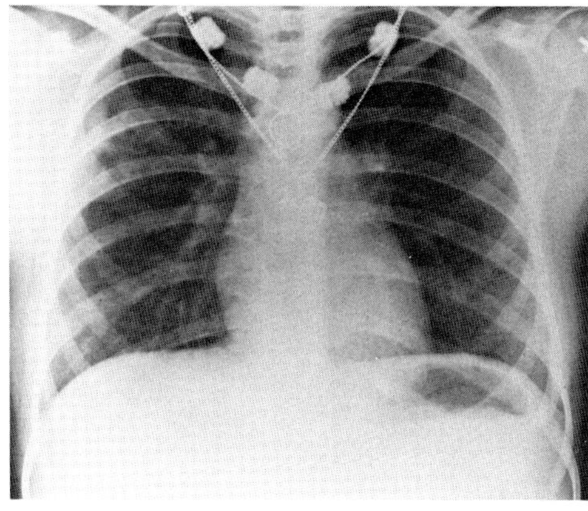

Figure 10-4. *Frontal radiograph of a 14-year-old diabetic with a 2-month history of fever and unproductive cough. A prior bronchoscopy had been unrevealing. Thoracoscopy and right upper lobe biopsy revealed* Cryptococcus neoformans *organisms.*

felt important to obtain multiple biopsy specimens from the pathologic area, not only from within the center of the lesion but also from around the periphery of the lesion, to define the complete spectrum of pathologic involvement. Usually, multiple specimens were obtained from within the same area in order to obtain tissue deep within the pulmonary parenchyma. This technique of multiple biopsies allowed a diagnostic accuracy of 93 percent in this group of patients. The single instance of failure to make an appropriate diagnosis was in a 2-month-old infant with pulmonary infiltrates in whom mechanical difficulties with the instruments precluded obtaining adequate biopsy specimens. Complications in the group of nonimmunosuppressed children were minimal, with a single instance of bleeding requiring transfusion.

Biopsy of Intrathoracic Tumors

In the past 5 years the proportion of children undergoing thoracoscopy for the diagnosis of intrathoracic tumors has increased. This technique has proven to be of exceptional value in these patients not only for tissue diagnosis but also for intrathoracic staging. A total of 24 procedures have been performed in 22 patients, ranging in age from 1 to 20 years (Table 10-4). In 9 patients the tumor was primarily parenchymal in location, as judged by preoperative chest roentgenograms. In 12 patients the lesion was mediastinal or intrapleural, and 3 patients underwent thoracoscopy for staging of known intrathoracic metastatic disease. In 12 (50 percent) of these procedures a diagnosis of intrathoracic malignancy was established by thoracoscopy. In two procedures, areas of unsuspected intrathoracic pathology were noted at the time of thoracoscopy (see Figure 31, p. vi), and this important information

Table 10-4
Thoracoscopy in Children with Tumors

Patients	22
Procedures	24
Ages	1–20 years
Accuracy	92%

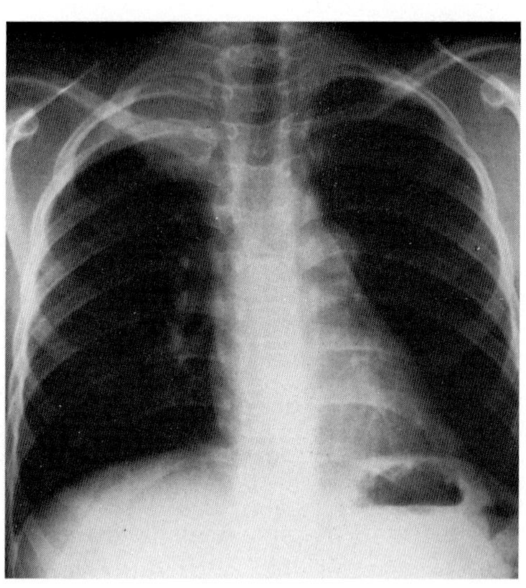

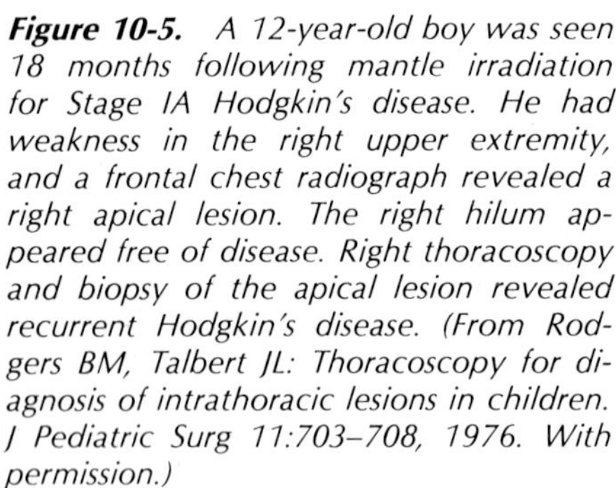

Figure 10-5. *A 12-year-old boy was seen 18 months following mantle irradiation for Stage IA Hodgkin's disease. He had weakness in the right upper extremity, and a frontal chest radiograph revealed a right apical lesion. The right hilum appeared free of disease. Right thoracoscopy and biopsy of the apical lesion revealed recurrent Hodgkin's disease. (From Rodgers BM, Talbert JL: Thoracoscopy for diagnosis of intrathoracic lesions in children. J Pediatric Surg 11:703–708, 1976. With permission.)*

allowed modification of subsequent therapy (Figure 10-5). The diagnostic accuracy of thoracoscopy in this entire group of patients was 92 percent. In 2 patients an inaccurate diagnosis was made by thoracoscopy: in both instances false-negative biopsy specimens were obtained. In one of these patients an intraparenchymal bronchogenic cyst was incorrectly diagnosed as a posterior mediastinal mass on the basis of chest roentgenograms, and the lesion could not be identified for biopsy at thoracoscopy (Figure 10-6). In a second patient, with suspicious mediastinal widening after therapy for Hodgkin's disease, a biopsy report of thymic tissue was obtained at thoracoscopy (Figure 10-7). With persistence of this enlargement, a tho-

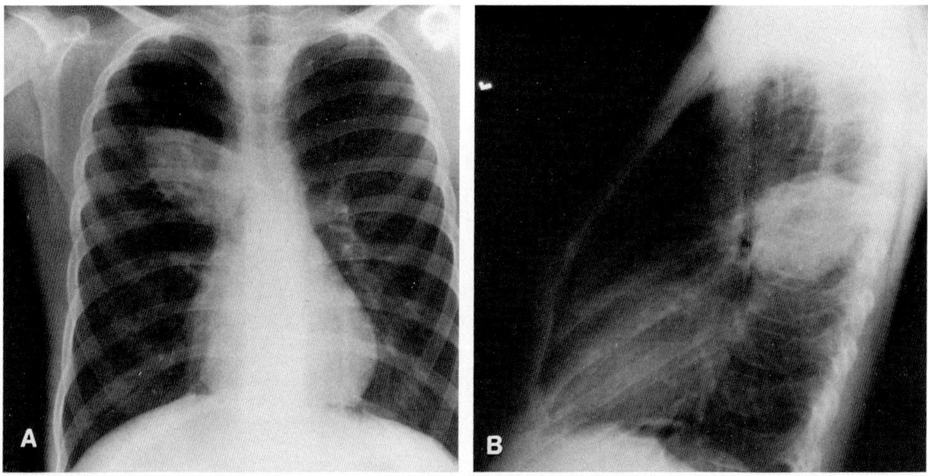

Figure 10-6. *Frontal and lateral chest radiographs of a 14-year-old boy with an asymptomatic mediastinal mass. The lesion was interpreted as being a pleural-based posterior mediastinal mass, probably neurogenic in origin. The posterior mediastinum appeared normal at thoracoscopy, and on thoracotomy this patient proved to have an intraparenchymal bronchogenic cyst. (From Rodgers BM, Moazam F, Talbert JL: Thoracoscopy in children. Ann Surg 189:176–180, 1979. With permission.)*

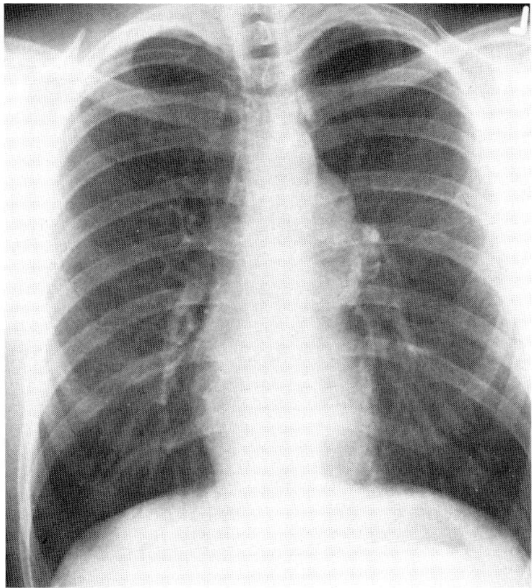

Figure 10-7. *Frontal chest radiograph of an 18-year-old boy 2 years following completion of chemotherapy for Stage IVA Hodgkin's disease. A persistent left mediastinal mass (arrows) was biopsied at thoracoscopy and contained only thymus. At thoracotomy 12 months later, a lymph node infiltrated with Hodgkin's disease was resected. (From Rodgers BM, Moazam F, Talbert JL: Thoracoscopy in children. Ann Surg 189:176–180, 1979. With permission.)*

racotomy was performed 12 months following thoracoscopy and a single mediastinal lymph node containing nodular sclerosing Hodgkin's disease was resected.

The complications of thoracoscopy procedures performed on patients with intrathoracic tumors have been minimal. There has been no instance of postoperative pneumothorax or bleeding in these patients. A single patient died within 30 days of the surgical procedure of pulmonary insufficiency secondary to extensive pulmonary metastases, an outcome unrelated to the surgical procedure.

Miscellaneous Therapeutic Procedures

Five patients have undergone thoracoscopy for various therapeutic reasons. The ages of these patients have ranged from 2 weeks to 17 years. Two older patients in this group have undergone thoracoscopy for treatment of pleural effusions. In one case, a malignant pleural effusion secondary to Hodgkin's disease was successfully treated with talc poudrage. In the other instance, a loculated post-traumatic pleural effusion was successfully evacuated. In three small infants, attempts were made to disrupt congenital pulmonary cysts causing respiratory embarassment (Figure 10-8).

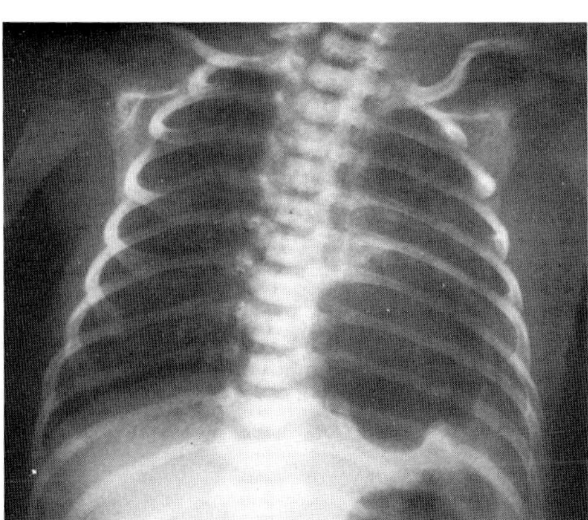

Figure 10-8. *Frontal chest radiograph of a 2-week-old infant with an enlarging left lower lobe pulmonary cyst. The wall of this cyst was successfully ruptured during thoracoscopy with complete evacuation of the cyst.*

In only one of these was this procedure successful. The technique of thoracoscopy is very difficult in infants under the age of 4–6 months. In these small children it is often impossible to achieve a sufficient pneumothorax to adequately visualize the intrathoracic structures. The rapid respiratory rate and relative noncompliance of the lung in these small infants hinders adequate pulmonary collapse. In view of these difficulties, this procedure should probably be reserved for patients older than 4 months of age, except in unusual circumstances.

Conclusion

The definitive diagnosis of intrathoracic diseases often presents a challenge to physicians involved in the care of pediatric patients. When both histopathologic and microbiologic examination of pulmonary tissue are required for therapeutic planning, the difficulties are greatly magnified. Successful management of many of these disorders requires an early and accurate diagnosis. The experience outlined in this review, as well as that of others, has indicated that the differential diagnosis of many of these pulmonary afflictions cannot reliably be made upon clinical or radiologic criteria alone. Although some of these illnesses, such as bacterial and fungal pneumonias, are infectious in origin and diagnoses may be made with simple aspiration procedures, many are from other causes, such as drug and radiation induced pneumonitis or neoplasms, and require tissue biopsy for diagnosis. Many of the procedures successfully used to obtain pulmonary tissue in adult patients, such as transbronchial pulmonary biopsy and transthoracic trephine biopsy, are not appropriate for use in small and uncooperative pediatric patients. Pulmonary needle aspiration has been used extensively in children with pulmonary infiltrates, but even in the most experienced hands, the diagnostic accuracy is disappointing, varying from 67 to 93 percent.[5,6] In addition, this procedure has not been without morbidity and even occasional mortality. The incidence of postaspiration pneumothorax has been reported as high as 57 percent, with approximately one-third of these patients requiring emergency insertion of an intercostal chest tube.[6] One of the most serious drawbacks of this procedure, however, has been the inability to obtain pulmonary tissue for meaningful histopathologic diagnosis in patients in whom specific microbiologic etiologies are not defined.[7,8] Because of the critical condition of many of these patients and the rapidity of progression of these processes, physicians have sought a safe technique with a high degree of accuracy for making these diagnoses with a single procedure. The standards that have evolved for children with pulmonary infiltrates or intrathoracic tumors have been open lung biopsy or a more extensive exploratory thoracotomy. These procedures are performed under general anesthesia, with endotracheal intubation, and the mortality with this approach in immunosuppressed patients with diffuse pulmonary involvement may be as high as 11–22 percent.[9] Many pediatricians are therefore hesitant to request open lung biopsy as a diagnostic modality early in the course of evaluating critically ill children, and frequently unnecessary delays in initiating specific therapy result.

Thoracoscopy, introduced by Jacobaeus in 1910, enjoyed considerable popularity in the early decades of this century for pleural lysis in patients with pulmonary tuberculosis undergoing therapeutic pneumothorax.[1] Because of inherent limitations in instrumentation and optics, the use of thoracoscopy became less prevalent with the rapid advances in thoracic surgery and anesthetic techniques. In the past decade the development of the Hopkins rod lens optical system has allowed production of sophisticated endoscopic equipment, sufficiently miniaturized for use in children. The availability of suitable instrumentation and the limitations of other available procedures indicated a need for a renewed trial of thoracoscopy for intrathoracic diagnosis. The data in this chapter indicate that the technique of thoracoscopy provides a very attractive alternative for the diagnosis of pulmonary parenchymal disease in both immunosuppressed and nonimmunosuppressed children. In 57 such procedures reported herein, the diagnostic accuracy has been 97 percent. The rapidity and safety of the thoracoscopy procedure has stimulated an early aggressive attitude toward the diagnosis of these pulmonary lesions and, we believe, has allowed for more effective therapy and improved survival in the immunosuppressed patients especially. In these patients, in whom an accurate and rapid diagnosis is essential for specific therapy, thoracoscopy has become the procedure of choice for obtaining pulmonary biopsy specimens. In comparison with other definitive diagnostic techniques useful in children, thoracoscopy appears to have a lesser morbidity and mortality. In these critically ill patients, this procedure can be performed rapidly with intravenous or regional block anesthetic techniques. Endotracheal intubation is not necessary and many postanesthetic respiratory complications are therefore avoided.

The technique of thoracoscopy offers several advantages over limited thoracotomy or needle biopsy techniques in children suspected of having intrathoracic tumors. Thoracoscopy may be performed in these patients with a minimum of morbidity and mortality. In addition, this technique allows for evaluation of the entire hemithorax and in some instances may allow detection of more distant areas of intrathoracic involvement. Selected biopsy specimens may be obtained from lesions in the mediastinum, pulmonary parenchyma, and chest wall, a capability not possible with a limited exploratory thoracotomy. The diagnostic accuracy of thoracoscopy in this group of patients has been 92 percent and has improved considerably with increasing experience with the technique and better anesthetic management. The addition of the stellate ganglion block has greatly facilitated the ability to retract the lung and visualize structures in the anterior mediastinum in these patients.

The attempts at using thoracoscopy as a therapeutic modality have had mixed results. The failures with therapeutic thoracoscopy in the small infants with pulmonary cysts probably reflect the very small size of these infants in whom a limited view within the hemithorax is possible. The technical difficulties of performing therapeutic thoracoscopy in these very small infants may lessen its usefulness in this age patient. Pleural lysis, on the other hand, is easily achieved through the thoracoscope, and further therapeutic indications in patients with loculated pleural effusions may evolve as our experience with this technique increases.

In summary, thoracoscopy has proven to be a safe and highly accurate method of obtaining intrathoracic biopsy specimens in children. With the use of small, rigid endoscopic telescopes and regional block anesthesia, a complete view of the contents of the hemithorax may be obtained and selective biopsies safely performed. The primary indications for the technique are for tissue diagnosis of pulmonary infiltrates in immunosuppressed or nonimmunosuppressed children and for diagnosis or staging of intrathoracic tumors.

References

1. Von Jacobaeus HC: Uber die Möglichkeit die Zystoskopie bei Untersuchung seröser Höhlungen anzuwenden. MMW 57:2090–2092, 1910
2. Brandt HJ, Mai J: Differential diagnosis of pleural effusion using thoracoscopy. Pneumonologie 145:192–203, 1971
3. DeCamp PT, Moseley PW, Scott ML, et al: Diagnostic thoracoscopy. Ann Thorac Surg 16:79–84, 1973
4. Lewis RJ, Kunderman PJ, Sisler GE, et al: Direct diagnostic thoracoscopy. Ann Thorac Surg 21:536–539, 1976
5. Chaudhary S, Hughes WT, Feldman S, et al: Percutaneous transthoracic needle aspiration of the lung: diagnosing *Pneumocystis carinii* pneumonitis. Am J Dis Child 131:902–907, 1977
6. Fontana RS, Miller WE, Beabout JW, et al: Transthoracic needle aspiration of discrete pulmonary lesions: experience in 100 cases. Med Clin North Am 54:961–971, 1970
7. Lincoln CP, Grover FL, Trinkle JK: Open versus needle biopsy of the lung. How valuable to the patient? J Thorac Cardiovasc Surg 69:507–509, 1975
8. Walzer PD, Perl DP, Krogstad DJ, et al: *Pneumocystis carinii* pneumonia in the United States: epidemiologic, diagnostic, and clinical features. Ann Intern Med 80:83–93, 1974
9. Michaelis LL, Leight GS, Powell RD, et al: Pneumocystis pneumonia: importance of early open lung biopsy. Ann Surg 183:301–306, 1976

The Technique of Laparoscopy

CHAPTER 11

Stephen L. Gans
Edward Austin

Laparoscopy, also known as peritoneoscopy, is the visualization of the peritoneal cavity and its contents by means of a telescope introduced through a tiny opening in the anterior abdominal wall after establishment of a pneumoperitoneum. The procedure has been done successfully for many years, reports appearing just after the turn of the century by Ott (in Petrograd), Kelling (in Dresden), and Jacobaeus (in Stockholm). Further investigations and developments were reported in the second decade by Bernheim, Nordentoeft, Tedesco, Renon, Rosenthal, Roccavilla, Schmidt, Johnsson, and Orndoff, using a variety of methods and makeshift instruments (the best of which appeared to be the Nitze cystoscope), some with and some without pneumoperitoneum. This historical background is well detailed by Cohen[1] in his monograph devoted mainly to the field of gynecology. He continues on to discuss the work and methods of later investigators and clinicians. Almost all of these efforts were made by gynecologists, gastroenterologists, and a few general surgeons, and were aimed for the most part at study of the conditions involved in gynecology and hepatology.

The use of laparoscopy in the pediatric age group was virtually unknown until we investigated the procedure and reported our initial methods and results in 1971[2] and further experience in 1973.[3] Since that time other investigators have confirmed our early results and laparoscopy is now an established method of investigation and treatment of a wide variety of conditions in infants and children. These events have become possible because of the technical developments in optics and illumination (see Chapter 1) that made possible miniature instruments with exceptional capability and performance.

This chapter is limited to a detailed description of methods and techniques; following chapters describe the wide applications and indications for their use.

It should be made clear at the outset that *laparoscopy is indicated for DIAGNOSIS only when more simple studies are not adequate and when exploratory laparotomy would therefore be considered. It is only indicated for THERAPY when such a procedure can be carried out safely without laparotomy.* The advantage of this technique is that it either avoids laparotomy altogether (which previously would have been indicated), or it establishes the need for operation.

In general, laparoscopy is contraindicated in infants and children for whom general anesthesia is contraindicated. It is further contraindicated in conditions where puncture of the abdominal wall might be hazardous. Such situations are peritonitis, intestinal obstructions, or where extensive scarring or adhesions are present from previous surgery.

Preparation

Laparoscopy is best carried out when the gastrointestinal tract is empty. Feedings should be withheld for an appropriate time depending upon the patient's age, and a cleansing enema can be used at an appropriate time if not contraindicated for any special reason. A nasogastric tube on suction will keep the stomach empty and the intestines from filling with swallowed air.

If the pelvic organs are to be examined, the bladder should be emptied. This should be checked by palpation under anesthesia, and preparations should be made for catheterization if the bladder obstructs the view necessary for a proper examination.

Anesthesia

Although in adults laparoscopy can sometimes be done under local anesthesia, general anesthesia with controlled respiration is necessary for infants and children because the pneumoperitoneum significantly inhibits diaphragmatic movement and, additionally, young patients are not able to cooperate well under these conditions. An exception is the unconscious patient with trauma, a situation described in Chapter 16. Experience has shown that with proper precautions, careful monitoring, and cooperative collaboration by the anesthesiologist, pneumoperitoneum does not impose undue strain on the respiratory or cardiovascular systems.

Equipment

We have used the Storz equipment* since the development of the Hopkins lens telescopes, and have found it to be complete and all-inclusive, well coordinated, efficient, and durable. The view obtained is unsurpassed, and photodocumentation is readily obtained. Other equipment and accessories are available from various sources.

Table 11-1 lists the instruments and apparatus suggested for examination, manipulation, and treatment. Figure 11-1 illustrates these instruments, and the following text describes how they are used.

*Karl Storz KG, Tuttlingen, West Germany; Storz Endoscopy–America, Culver City, California.

Table 11-1
Equipment for Pediatric Laparoscopy: Sterile Setup
(See Figure 11-1)

For Examination	
A.	Pointed knife, No. 11 blade
B.	Mosquito hemostats, straight and curved
C.	Veress pneumoperitoneum needle, pediatric size, 70 mm
D.	Syringe, 10 ml, and normal saline, 50 ml
E.	CO_2 insufflation tubing
F.	Examining trocar and cannula, O.D. 5 mm
G.	Hopkins forward-oblique telescope, 30°
H.	Fiberoptic light cable
*	Teaching attachment
For Further Manipulation or Instrumentation	
I.	Long needle for injection
*	Liver biopsy needle, optional choice
J.	Trocar and cannula, O.D. 4 mm, for manipulating instruments
K.	Palpation probe
L.	Biopsy forceps
M.	Grasping forceps
N.	Suction-coagulation cannula probe
*	Cable to connect above to electrosurgical unit
O.	Desufflation key
P.	Spare parts (gaskets, washers)
*	Sponges, skin suture, needle holder, and scissors
Alternate to C, F, and G above	
	(See Figure 11-6A, B, Gans-Austin single puncture pediatric laparoscope)
Accessory Equipment (not sterile)	
*	Gas insufflator
*	Light source
*	Electrosurgical unit

*Not shown in Figure 11-1.

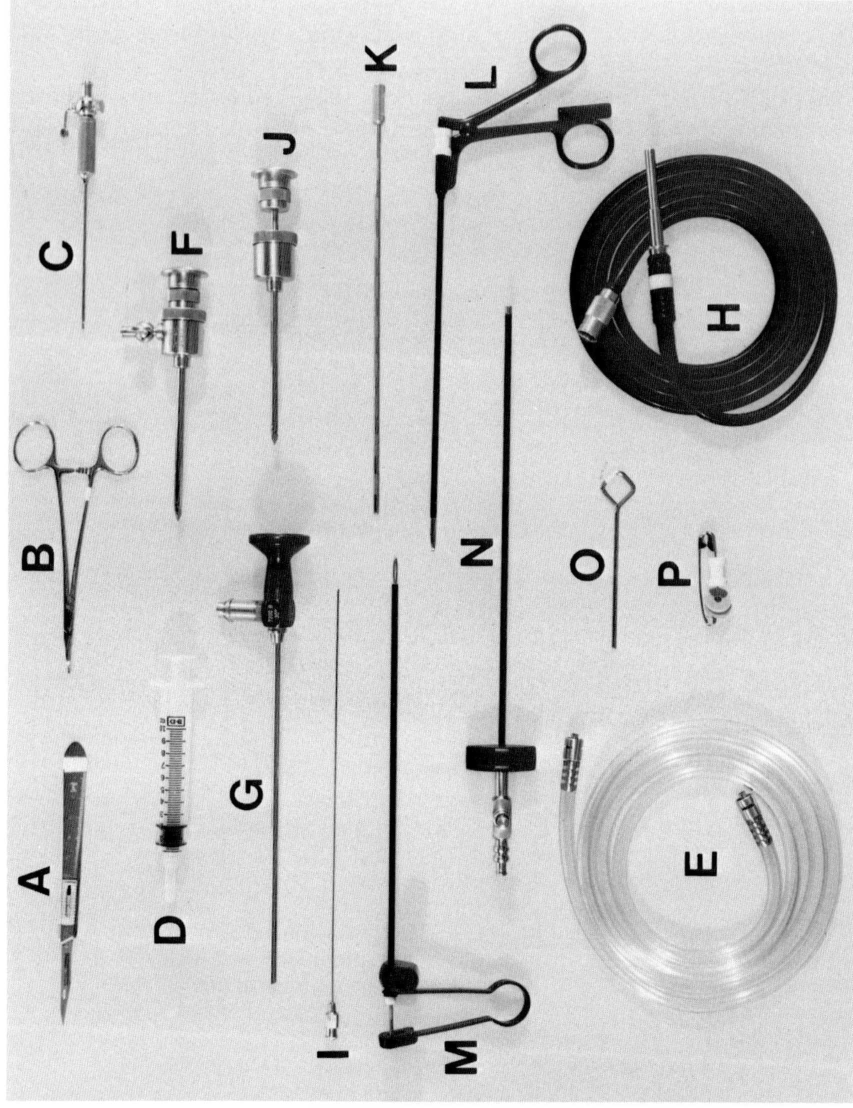

Figure 11-1. *Recommended sterile equipment for pediatric laparoscopy. See Table 11-1.*

Technique

Under satisfactory endotracheal anesthesia with the patient in the supine position on the operating table, with a secure intravenous running and with cardiac, respiratory, and temperature monitors in use, the skin of the lower chest and the entire abdomen is prepared and draped. The operating team and equipment are appropriately positioned (Figure 11-2).

The initial puncture of the abdomen is usually made around the rim of the umbilicus for three reasons: it is easiest to perform here because of the thinness of the abdominal wall; the central location permits examination of the entire peritoneal cavity, at least in an infant or child; and it leaves an almost invisible scar. The upper or lower rim is chosen depending upon whether the prime target is the upper or lower abdomen. Exceptions are the neonate and the small or malnourished infant. Here the tissues around the umbilicus are too thin and air will leak out, making it more difficult to maintain the pneumoperitoneum. In such patients we puncture the abdomen through the medial portion of one of the rectus muscles, above or below the level of the umbilicus, mindful of the presence of the epigastric vessels.

A stab wound is made in the skin with the pointed knife blade. The abdominal wall is tented up by the operator and assistant by grasping it, above and below, using a sponge between the fingers to aid in maintaining traction, and the needle with the spring-controlled blunt stylet is introduced into the peritoneal cavity. As this needle pierces the peritoneum, the blunt stylet springs out, thus protecting the abdominal contents from injury by further advancement (Figure 11-3). The needle is

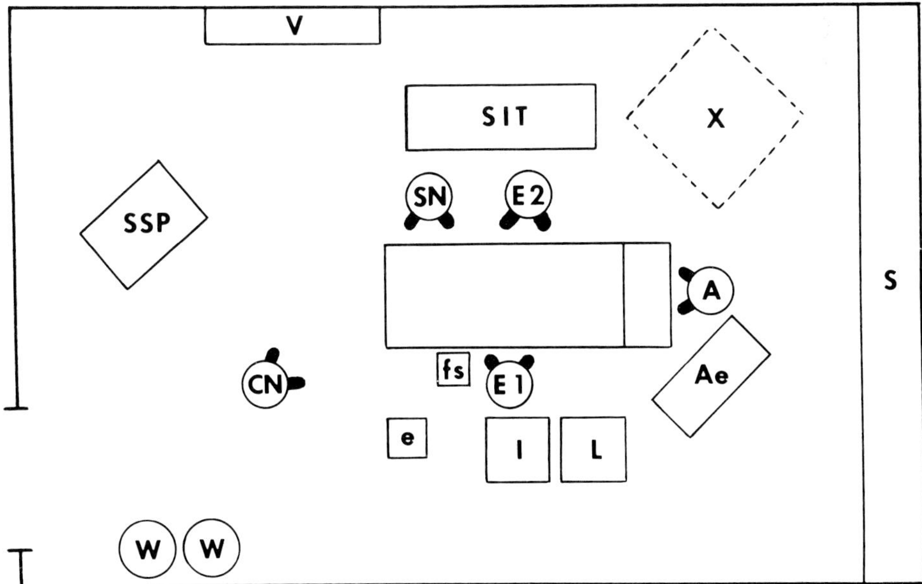

Figure 11-2. *Position of personnel and equipment for pediatric laparoscopy. (A) anesthesiologist; (E1) endoscopist; (E2) assistant; (SN) scrub nurse; (CN) circulating nurse; (Ae) anesthesia equipment; (I)* CO_2 *insufflator; (L) light source; (e) electrocoagulation unit, with (fs) foot switch; (SIT) sterile instrument table; (SSP) sterile spare parts; (S) storage; (V) x-ray view box; (W) waste cans; (X) x-ray equipment (desirable).*

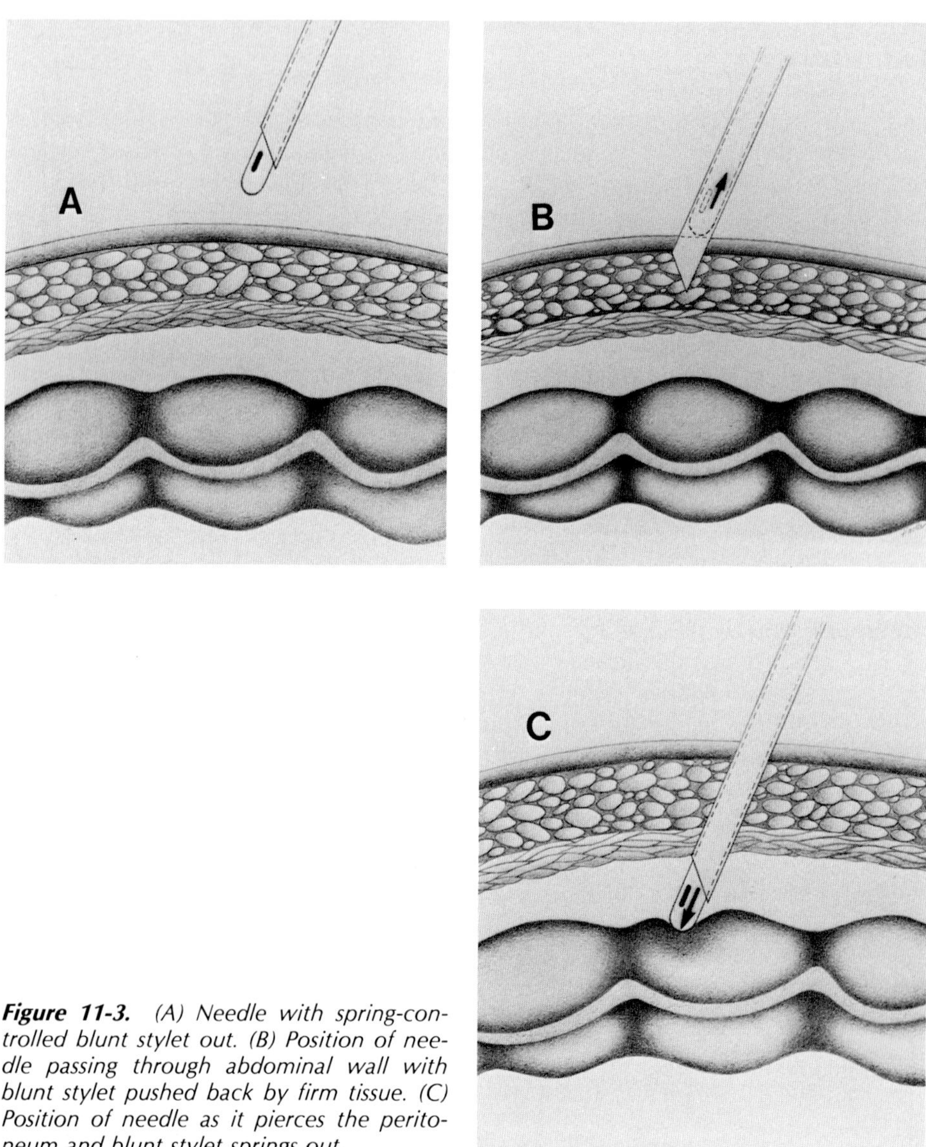

Figure 11-3. *(A) Needle with spring-controlled blunt stylet out. (B) Position of needle passing through abdominal wall with blunt stylet pushed back by firm tissue. (C) Position of needle as it pierces the peritoneum and blunt stylet springs out.*

tested by side-to-side motion to see if the intra-abdominal portion moves freely. A 10-ml syringe is connected to the needle and aspiration is carried out to assure that no bowel contents are present in the needle. Five to 10 ml of saline are injected to demonstrate free flow.

Pneumoperitoneum is initiated by connecting the needle to a carbon dioxide cylinder and an insufflating device that can control flow and pressure as desired, or automatically when so adjusted and set (Figure 11-4). Carbon dioxide is used because it is rapidly absorbed and excreted, and it does not support combustion. Abdominal pressure in an infant should not exceed 10–15 mm Hg. In neonates or infants it is very important that the insufflation proceed slowly, with careful monitoring of the patient by the anesthesiologist.

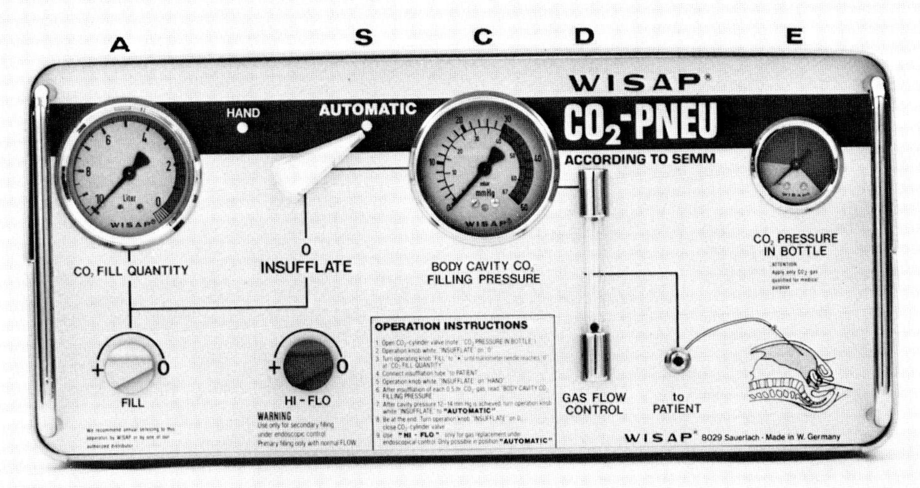

Figure 11-4. *Insufflating apparatus. Letter A shows the CO_2 fill quantity; S is the switch from manual to automatic control; C is the gauge that monitors intraperitoneal pressure; D is a flow indicator; and E indicates the CO_2 pressure in the cylinder.*

During insufflation the abdomen is gently percussed and palpated with the fingers and when the pneumoperitoneum is considered adequate, the needle is removed.* The skin nick is enlarged by spreading with a hemostat until it can snugly admit the 5-mm (O.D.) cannula. The abdominal wall is again tented up by the operator and the assistant by grasping it above and below the puncture, and the cannula with a pointed trocar is then directed with a twisting motion through the abdominal wall and into the intraperitoneal air cushion.

The trocar is then removed and replaced with the appropriate telescope (Figure 11-5). Carbon dioxide does not escape because of a valve in the cannula. Inspection of the peritoneal contents may now begin. Those who see this procedure performed for the first time are usually amazed at the clear panorama, and even more so by the enlarged and detailed closeup view. Fogging of the telescope end may be prevented by prewarming the instrument and by the use of an antifog solution (see pp. 51–52). Should fogging occur, it may be simply and easily cleared by gently touching the bowel wall with the telescope end.

Needle biopsy or injection can be performed through a second puncture in direct view of the telescope. For more involved procedures, a second trocar and cannula (O.D. 4 mm) is introduced through a separate nick and puncture in an appropriate location for the projected manipulation, the point of this trocar and cannula appearing in the peritoneal cavity in direct view of the examining telescope (Figure 11-5). The trocar is removed and through this cannula a variety of instruments can be introduced. These include a palpating probe, biopsy forceps, grasping forceps, and a combined suction and electrocoagulation device (see Figure 11-1). The indications and use of these instruments are described in subsequent chapters.

---

*Compare the procedure at this point with the procedure described on page 158, in which the single puncture instrument and technique are used.

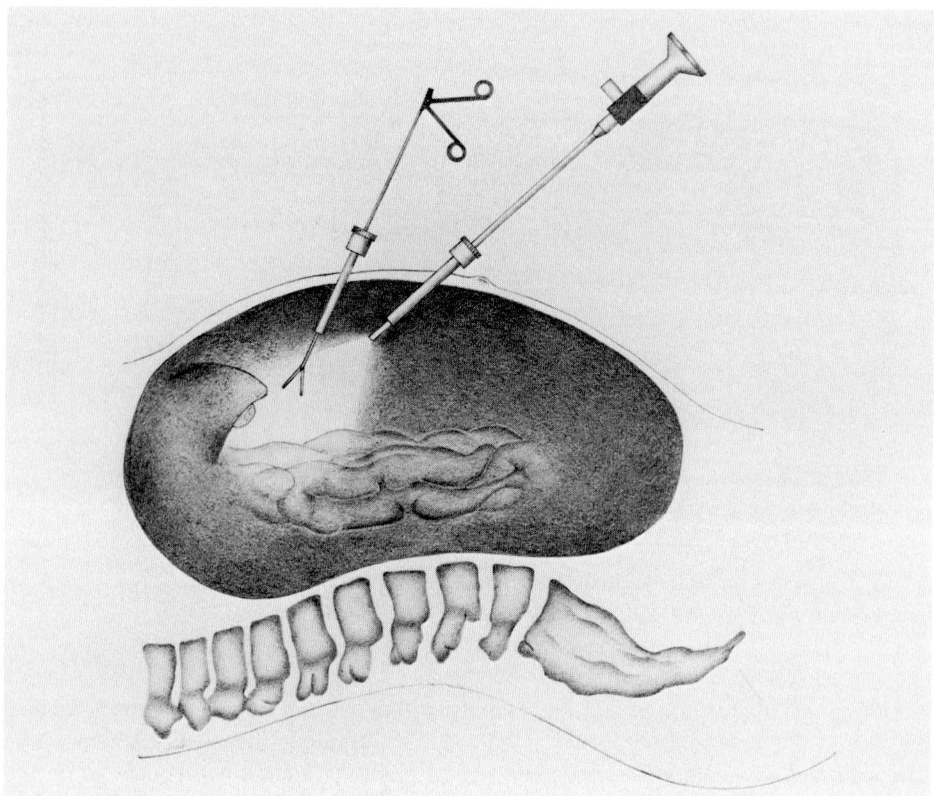

Figure 11-5. *Diagram of pneumoperitoneum and telescope inserted through a cannula near the umbilicus for inspection of the upper peritoneal contents. A second cannula has been inserted through which a manipulating instrument has been introduced. Valves in the cannulas prevent the escape of gas.*

An alternative method for examination is the single puncture technique. A special instrument (Figure 11-6) combines a somewhat larger Veress needle with a cannula so that they are introduced simultaneously in the same manner as described on pages 155 and 156 for introduction of the Veress needle alone. When pneumoperitoneum is adequate, the Veress needle is removed, leaving the cannula in position, and a telescope is inserted through this cannula. This method obviates the need for a second blind puncture with a trocar and cannula.

At the conclusion of the procedure, the gas is allowed to escape by opening the valve in the cannula with a special key. The skin edges of the puncture wounds are approximated with appropriate sutures.

Complications

We have now carried out more than 300 laparoscopies without complication. This testifies to the safety of this procedure when performed with proper precautions. We are aware of two serious complications that occur rarely and indicate laparoto-

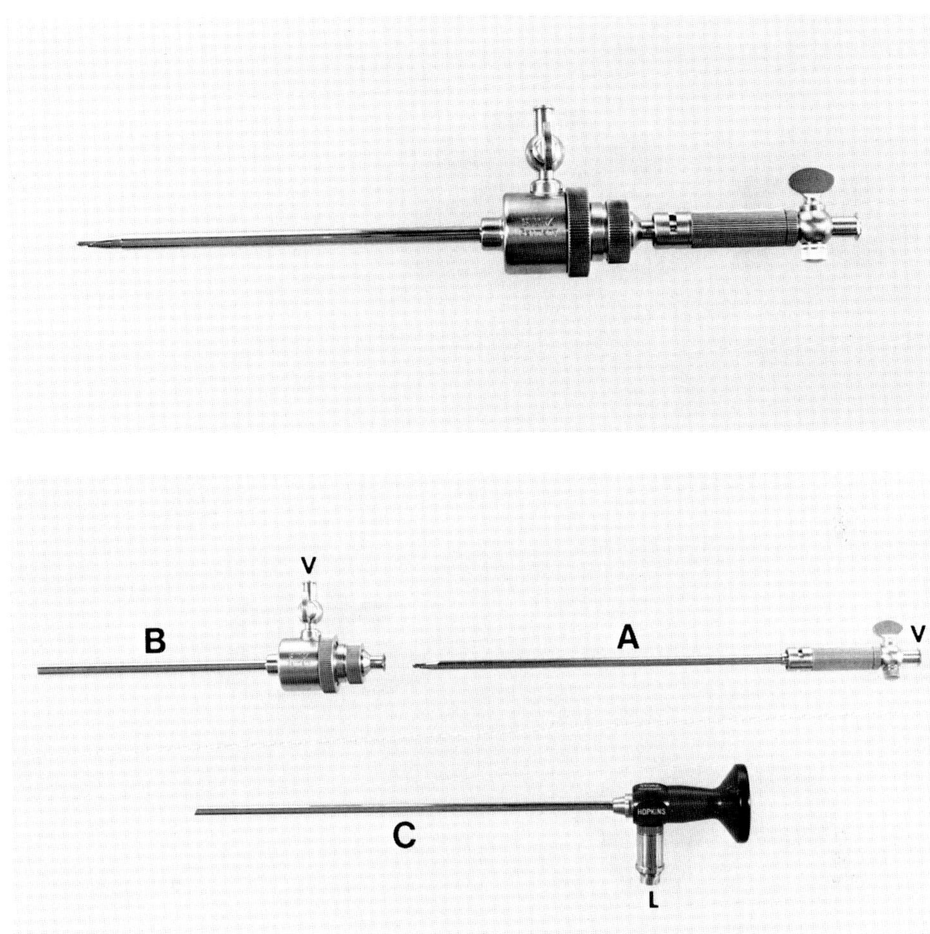

Figure 11-6. *(Top) Gans-Austin single puncture laparoscope, assembled and ready for introduction. (Bottom) (A) Needle with spring-controlled blunt stylet and valve connection (V) for introduction of CO_2, withdrawn from (B) cannula, also with valve connection (V) for insufflation of CO_2 during examination and equipped with inner valve to prevent escape of pneumoperitoneum gas. (C) Hopkins forward-oblique telescope, 30°, O.D. 4 mm.*

my for correction. One is perforation of the bowel during blind puncture of the abdominal wall, or by inadvertent use of manipulating instruments or electrocoagulation. The other is uncontrollable bleeding from a biopsy site. Both of these complications are readily identified through the laparoscope at the time of occurrence, and proper surgical therapy is carried out. The incidence of these complications is not accurately known, but it must be very small, being entirely absent in several large series of cases.

When one considers that laparoscopy is only done when laparotomy is the alternative, and that such laparoscopy very often avoids laparotomy, the low risk of this procedure is acceptable when proper indications and precautions are used.

References

1. Cohen MR: Laparoscopy, Culdoscopy and Gynecography. Philadelphia, Saunders, 1970, chap 2. Historical background, p 6
2. Gans SL, Berci G: Advances in endoscopy of infants and children. J Pediatr Surg 6:199–233, 1971
3. Gans SL, Berci G: Peritoneoscopy in infants and children. J Pediatr Surg 8:399–405, 1973

Laparoscopy in Hepatology and Hepatobiliary Diseases

CHAPTER 12

Urs G. Stauffer

In 1971 we in the Department of Pediatric Surgery, University Children's Hospital, Zurich started to use laparoscopic techniques. During the first few years laparoscopy was performed mainly to help with the diagnosis of general metabolic and liver diseases and for exact evaluation of the inner genitalia in congenital malformations of the urogenital tract. Since then many other indications for laparoscopy have emerged. Today we use diagnostic laparoscopic techniques in cases of cholestatic icterus, suspected intra-abdominal tumors, especially primary and secondary liver tumors, but also in cases of undiagnosed abdominal pain, suspected atypical appendicitis,[1] and occasionally in children with blunt abdominal trauma. In some cases the laparoscope has also been found useful in placing peritoneal dialysis catheters under direct vision.[2]

Between 1971 and 1980 a total of 149 laparoscopies were carried out. The indications are listed in Table 12-1. The youngest child to undergo laparoscopy was 5 days, the oldest 16 years old. All laparoscopies were performed under general anesthesia and intubation.[2,3] (See the general techniques for laparoscopy described in Chapter 11.)

In this chapter we discuss the indications for laparoscopy in hepatology and hepatobiliary diseases with special reference to our own experience in 85 cases. The

Table 12-1
Indications for Laparoscopy in 149 Patients*

Hepatology and hepatobiliary diseases	85
Malformations of the urogenital tract	32
Abdominal pain	25
Blunt abdominal trauma	4
Placing of peritoneal catheters for dialysis	3
Total	149

*University Children's Hospital, Zurich, 1971–1980

indications for laparoscopy in these 85 patients are listed in Table 12-2. The advantages of laparoscopy compared with needle biopsies and exploratory laparotomy, respectively, are described. Some special additional techniques in laparoscopic investigations in hepatobiliary atresia will shortly be mentioned.

Advantages of Laparoscopy in Liver Biopsy

Hepatobiliary conditions include a group of categories with a wide variety of patients who, after thorough study, may still require biopsy of a piece of liver tissue for accurate diagnosis.

Undoubtedly the simplest method of liver biopsy is with a percutaneous needle. The hazards are few when the contraindications are respected, and the results in general are satisfactory. When this is not the case and open operation for liver biopsy might be considered, however, our experience has shown that laparoscopic examination and biopsy have distinct advantages over both blind needle biopsy and open laparotomy.

Upon laparoscopic examination the color, size, structure, and feel of the liver can be evaluated and the presence of cysts, hemangiomas, nodules, tumors, or diffuse hepatic involvement noted before the biopsy needle or biopsy forceps is directed under clear vision into the most promising areas. Focal or nodular lesions can be missed by blind needling, and direct observation is a safety factor in preventing

Table 12-2
Laparoscopy in Hepatology and Hepatobiliary Diseases: Indications in 85 Patients*

Metabolic diseases (with involvement of the liver)	51
Cholestatic icterus	25
Liver tumors (primary and secondary)	5
Miscellaneous	4
Total	85

*University Children's Hospital, Zurich, 1971–1980

penetration of vascular or other potentially harmful targets. Lesions of pinhead size can be accurately biopsied with ease. If bleeding or leakage of bile persists after biopsy, it is readily observed and controlled by electrocoagulation. When indicated, relatively large pieces of liver tissue can be removed for histologic, electron-microscopic, and biochemical investigations. The spleen as well can be observed if desired.

Laparoscopy Compared with Exploratory Laparotomy

When a laparoscopy is performed, the whole abdominal cavity and most intra-abdominal organs can be inspected, which is usually not possible through a small exploratory laparotomy. Animal experiments that we have performed have shown that adhesions following laparoscopy occur much less commonly than after exploratory laparotomy; this has also been noted in the literature. In most cases we have seen no adhesion formation at all. This allows the taking of repeated biopsy specimens through the laparoscope in order to control the course of a given disease and avoid the danger of a possible adhesive obstruction, which may occur after exploratory laparotomy at any time. A further advantage of laparoscopy is that it does not take as much time as exploratory laparotomy. Liver biopsies performed through the laparoscope hardly take more than 10–20 minutes in the hands of an experienced operator. Following laparoscopy children can be discharged from the hospital within 24 hours. The time of hospitalization is thus markedly shorter with this technique than with exploratory laparotomy. Finally it must be added that the parents of our young patients have the impression that laparoscopy is a much smaller and less severe undertaking than laparotomy, especially as the abdominal scar that is left is hardly visible.

Contraindications

An important contraindication to laparoscopy is the presence of intra-abdominal adhesions, especially those secondary to previous laparotomies and intestinal obstructions. In these cases there may be an increased danger of intestinal perforation or hemorrhage. We also do not advise laparoscopy in cases of generalized peritonitis. The procedure is contraindicated in patients with disturbances of blood coagulation, especially those on anticoagulant treatment or patients with thrombocytopenia of less than 30,000/mm^3.

Complications

There have been no complications (such as hemorrhage, intestinal perforation, peritonitis, and so forth) in any of the 149 children who have undergone laparoscopy in the past 10 years in our department. All patients who had a purely diagnostic biopsy performed could be discharged on the next day. Several complications have, however, been described in the literature.[4–10]

Metabolic Diseases

Since 1971 we have routinely performed laparoscopy in cases of metabolic diseases involving the liver. Compared with the blind needle biopsy there are many advantages (which have been discussed previously).

Technique of Laparoscopy

The laparoscope is inserted in the usual place, just beneath the umbilicus (see Chapter 11). The abdominal cavity is inspected and an additional minute incision is made with a pointed knife midway between the umbilicus and the left anterior iliac spine. A small trocar and cannula are inserted through this incision into the abdominal cavity and the biopsy forceps is passed through the cannula. The biopsy can now be taken under direct vision. If necessary, the site of the biopsy can be coagulated with the aid of electrocoagulation applied to the biopsy forceps or with the suction-coagulation instrument. As reliable enzyme diagnosis of the liver can only be carried out on adequately sized specimens we usually take at least two biopsies. These are immediately handed to the pathologist and electronmicroscopy specialist or biochemist in the operating theater. It must be added that hemorrhage from the biopsies is usually negligible.

Case Material

Between 1971 and 1980 laparoscopy and liver biopsies were performed on 51 children with suspected metabolic diseases. The different diagnoses in this group of patients are summarized in Table 12-3. In 3 children a suspected congenital metabolic disturbance was excluded.

Table 12-3
Diagnosis in 51 Patients with Metabolic Diseases Involving the Liver

Diagnosis	No.
Glycogenoses	
Type I	9
Type II	1
Type IV	1
Hereditary fructose intolerance	11
Fructose-1, 6-diphosphatase deficiency	2
Lysosomal storage disease	6
Lipid storage disease	7
Normal histology	3
Various (mucopolysaccharidosis, Wilson's disease, α-1-antitrypsin deficiency, Niemann-Pick disease)	11
Total	51

Cholestatic Icterus

Cholestatic Icterus in Newborn and Young Infants

About half of the children who were laparoscoped for cholestatic icterus were infants between 1 and 4 months of age. A definite differential diagnosis between neonatal hepatitis and biliary atresia is rarely possible on the basis of clinical or laboratory findings.[2,11,12] In our experience this problem has been greatly facilitated by the use of the laparoscope.

Technique

After a general inspection of the abdominal cavity and inspection of the surface of the liver the falciform ligament is followed from the umbilicus to the liver, and the undersurface of the liver on the right side of the ligament is inspected in order to find the gallbladder. If a gallbladder is present, a Veress needle is inserted through the abdominal wall and liver parenchyma into the gallbladder under direct vision (Figure 12-1A). The indirect puncture of the gallbladder via the liver avoids the possibility of a subsequent biliary peritonitis. Radiopaque contrast material is then injected through the Veress needle; if the resulting cholangiogram shows an intact extrahepatic biliary system and if there is free flow of the dye into the duodenum, the examination can be discontinued (Figure 12-1B). If, however, no gallbladder or only a rudimentary gallbladder can be observed or if the extrahepatic biliary system can be only partly visualized (e.g., if there is no hepatic duct (Figure 12-1C), or a reflux into the large intrahepatic branches of the biliary system is not

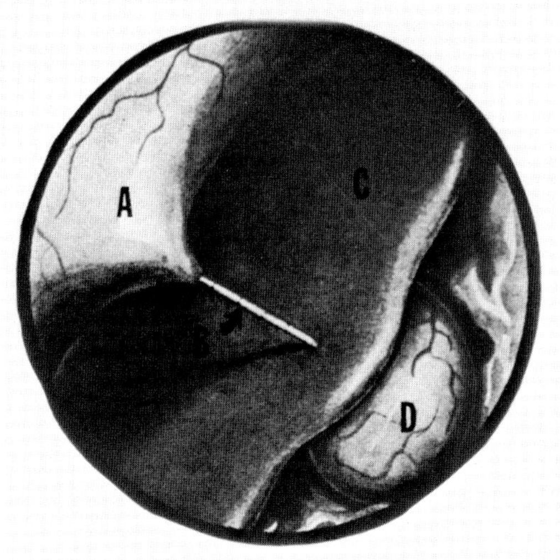

Figure 12-1A. *Transcutaneous transhepatic cholangiography under laparoscopic control. (A) Abdominal wall. (B) Needle or Teflon catheter. (C) Liver. (D) Gallbladder.*

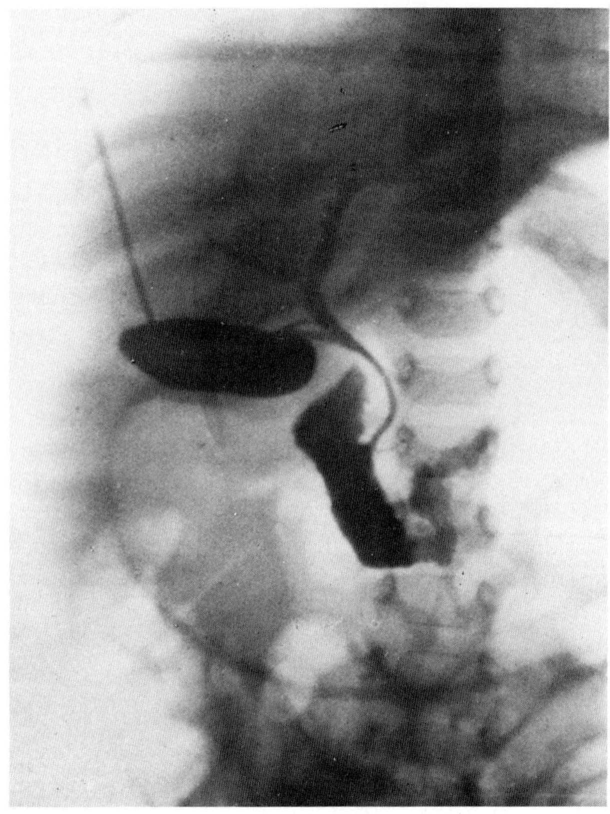

Figure 12-1B. *Normal biliary system. Good drainage into the duodenum, and good backflow into the liver.*

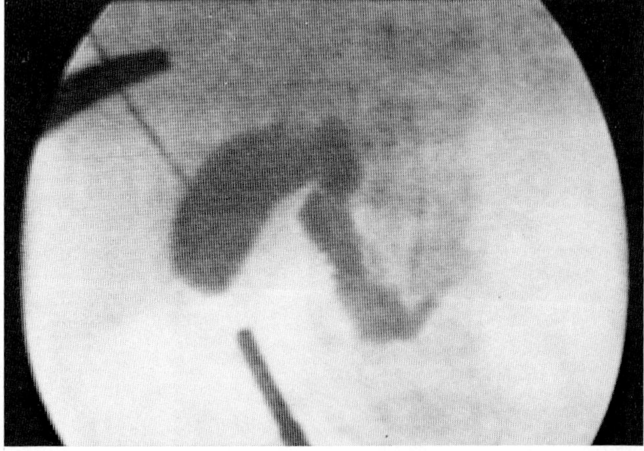

Figure 12-1C. *Proximal biliary atresia. Only the gallbladder and distal duct are filled with dye.*

Table 12-4
Diagnosis of 25 Patients with Cholestatic Icterus

Neonatal hepatitis	7
Biliary atresia	5
Choledochal cyst	1
Chronic hepatitis	4
Subacute hepatitis	1
Cholestatic icterus of unknown etiology	2
Cirrhosis of the liver	
Secondary to malaria	1
Secondary to Hodgkin's disease	2
Secondary to xanthomatous disease	1
Unknown etiology	1
Total	25

observed), a laparotomy should be carried out during the same anesthesia and, if necessary, surgical correction performed.[2,11,12]

Cholestatic Icterus in Infants and Children

In all infants and children with cholestatic icterus, laparoscopy and liver biopsy play an important part in the diagnosis and prognosis mainly of subacute or chronic inflammatory liver diseases and in cases of progressive cirrhosis (see Table 12-4).

Case Material

Between 1971 and 1980 laparoscopy with liver biopsy was performed on a total of 25 children with cholestatic icterus. Thirteen of these patients were infants under the age of 4 months with suspected extrahepatic biliary atresia. In 5 children where an extrahepatic biliary atresia was found, and in 1 child where a choledochal cyst was present, hepatoportoenterostomy was performed under the same anesthesia. The other children were between 6 months and 14 years of age. These were mainly children with chronic hepatitis and cirrhosis of different origins. The laparoscopic diagnoses of all 25 patients can be seen in Table 12-4.

Primary and Secondary Liver Tumors

In cases of abdominal tumors where the pathologic process is in doubt and where there is a possibility that the tumors arise from the liver, or where there is a possibility of liver metastases, laparoscopy can be most helpful. Five children were subjected to laparoscopy to determine whether they had a primary or a secondary liver tumor. In one 8-year-old boy a primary liver carcinoma was discovered (see Figure 32, p. vi). In 2 other patients solitary liver metastases (secondary to an orchioblastoma and to a neuroblastoma, respectively) were seen. In another patient the extent of a lymphosarcoma of the small intestine could be evaluated. In a

4-year-old girl with an apparent liver tumor the size of the child's head, a retroperitoneal chylus cyst was discovered and excised under the same anesthesia.

Conclusion

Today laparoscopy is an essential tool in the diagnosis of hepatic and hepatobiliary diseases in infancy and childhood. The many advantages compared with exploratory laparotomy and needle puncture have been described and discussed. We have not encountered any complications in our series of 85 patients with laparoscopy, laparoscopic liver biopsy, and transhepatic cholangiography. It must, however, be stressed that these techniques should only be carried out by those experienced in this type of investigation.

References

1. Schwobël MG, Stauffer UG: Der Stellenwert der Laparoskopie bei Verdacht auf akute Appendizitis. Z Kinderchir 29(1):24–29, 1980
2. Stauffer UG, Hirsig J: Unsere Erfahrungen mit der Laparoskopie bei Säuglingen und Kindern. Z Kinderchir suppl 27:134–137, 1979
3. Dangel P: Indikation, Technik und Gefahren der Narkose im Rahmen endoskopischer Untersuchungen bei Kindern. Z Kinderchir suppl 27:14–23, 1979
4. Cohen R: Laparoscopy, Culdoscopy and Gynecography. Philadelphia, Saunders, 1970, p 42
5. Mosenthal WT: Peritonescopy. Am J Surg 123:421, 1972
6. Frangenheim H: Die Stellung der Laparoskopie bei gynäkologischen und chirurgischen Problemen im Kindesalter, in Rossi E (ed): Pädiatrische Fortbildungskurse für die Praxis (vol 39). New York, Basel, 1974, p 71
7. Prim DV: Ruptured spleen as a complication of laparoscopy and pelvic laparotomy. Report of an unusual complication. Am J Obstet Gynecol 7:983, 1974
8. Milliken RA, Milliken GM: Gastric perforation. Rare complication of laparoscopy. NY State J Med 1:77, 1975
9. Alfonsin AE, Chaudet A: Mobilidad en laparoscopía. Obstet Ginecol Latinoam 3/4:102, 1974
10. Brindle GF, Soliman MG: Anaesthetic complications in surgical outpatients. Can Anaesth Soc J 5:613, 1975
11. Stauffer UG, Hirsig J: Kongenitale Gallengangsatresie, in Bettex M, Genton N, Stockmann M, (eds): Lehrbuch der Kinderchirurgie, begründet von M. Grob (ed 2). Stuttgart/New York, Georg Thieme Verlag, 1982, pp 178–192
12. Cook RCM, Rickham PP: The Liver and biliary tract, in Rickham PP, Lister J, Irving IM (eds): Neonatal Surgery (ed 2). London/Boston, Butterworths, 1978, pp 483–500

Laparoscopy for Gynecologic Disorders

CHAPTER 13

Lucian L. Leape

Laparoscopy was developed as a diagnostic and therapeutic modality in large measure by adult gynecologists in Europe. Indeed, by far the greatest application of laparoscopy has been in gynecologic practice, where it has probably become the most frequently performed invasive gynecologic procedure. Laparoscopy has become accepted as the primary method of tubal interruption for sterilization and has also been of value in the assessment and treatment of many other gynecologic problems.

In children, use of laparoscopy should be considered any time there is a question of the status of the uterus, tubes, and ovaries, regardless of the age of the patient. In practice it will find greatest application at three different ages: in the newborn with ambiguous genitalia, in the young girl with precocious puberty, and in the adolescent postpubertal female.

The Neonate with Ambiguous Genitalia (Intersex)

Few things are more distressing to parents than a question of gender assignment in a newborn infant. Because of this, the newborn with ambiguous genitalia represents an emergency every bit as serious psychosocially as a congenital diaphragmatic hernia is physically. It is the physician's responsibility to determine the sex assignment as rapidly as possible. Fortunately, methods now exist that make this possible in a matter of hours, not days. Laparoscopy can help obviate the need for laparotomy in some of these infants.[1]

Gender assignment in large measure depends on functional anatomy, even if this conflicts with genetic or gonadal sex. In most patients a careful physical examination, a buccal smear for chromatin bodies, and a sinogram to delineate a urogenital sinus or vagina will give adequate information for prompt assignment. In some infants with ambiguous genitalia, particularly those in whom there is a question of gonadal dysgenesis or true hermaphroditism, it is essential to obtain a gonadal biopsy and desirable to assess whether there is a uterus present. It is in these patients that laparoscopy is useful.

Laparoscopy should be performed under general anesthesia in all infants and children, including newborn infants. After induction of anesthesia, sinusoscopy will give detailed information regarding the status of the urogenital sinus, the opening of the urethra, and whether there is a cervix present. Laparoscopy may then be carried out in the usual fashion. It is safer to perform the pneumoperitoneum by hand injection of carbon dioxide gas with a syringe to avoid overdistention or extreme variations in pressure.

The presence (or absence) of the uterus, tubes, and ovaries can usually be readily established. Biopsy of the gonads is usually best done through a separate cannula introduced laterally low in the abdomen. If only "streak" gonads are found, consideration must be given to their removal. Otherwise, biopsy will provide guidance in terms of future management. Vaginoplasty and clitoral recession can be done under the same anesthetic or may be deferred until the patient is a month or two of age. It is essential that these patients have long-term followup, because mechanical abnormalities of the uterus may not show up until puberty.

Precocious Puberty

Early breast development and the appearance of pubic hair in the young child is a distressing phenomenon, one that deserves prompt and thorough evaluation. Abnormalities of the ovary, adrenal, and pituitary must be systematically sought and excluded. If diagnostic studies fail to reveal a pituitary or adrenal cause of early puberty, ovarian biopsy is essential. Laparoscopy permits ovarian assessment, including biopsy, without the need for laparotomy. Some patients will be found to have an ovarian tumor. If so, surgical excision under the same anesthetic is indicated. In most, however, the ovary will appear normal or somewhat enlarged. Biopsy may then reveal evidence of gonadotropic stimulation, idiopathic precocity, the most common cause.[2] If there is a luteinizing cyst, aspiration and fenestration laparoscopically may be curative, although cystectomy may be required.

Adolescent Gynecologic Disorders

Gynecologic abnormalities are not rare in adolescents, and the postpubertal teenager is susceptible to most of the afflictions of adult women: dysmenorrhea, dyspareunia, abnormalities of pregnancy, and pelvic pain. In addition, congenital abnormalities of the generative organs may first become manifest at puberty by amenorrhea, cyclic pelvic pain, or the occurrence of a pelvic mass.

Amenorrhea

Primary amenorrhea requires an extensive evaluation, including biochemical assessment of pituitary and ovarian function. Laparoscopy may be indicated to determine if there are uterine abnormalities such as hypoplasia, agenesis, or intrauterine or high vaginal septa.[3] Blockage of uterine drainage from a congenital malformation is usually associated with palpable enlargement of the uterus and cyclic pain due to retained menstruum. Ovarian abnormalities such as polycystic malformation may also be diagnosed and confirmed by laparoscopy. In secondary amenorrhea, diagnosis and biopsy of Stein-Levinthal ovaries may be carried out by laparoscopy.

Gonadal Dysplasia

In patients with Turner's syndrome laparoscopy may be of value in assessing the condition of the dysplastic ovaries so as to predict the need for estrogen therapy.[2]

Pelvic Pain

Lower abdominal or pelvic pain is not rare in adolescent postpubertal girls and may be very difficult to treat. Endometriosis can become manifest within months after menarche. Laparoscopy is the easiest way to make the diagnosis, and peritoneal implants may be biopsied for confirmation.[4] Ovarian and paraovarian cysts, as well as abnormalities of the uterus and tubes, may be the cause of recurring pelvic pain. Most can be readily diagnosed, and often treated as well, laparoscopically[5] (see Figure 33, p. vi).

In the sexually active young woman pelvic inflammatory disease must be considered. This diagnosis is also difficult to prove, for cultures are more often negative than positive. Even a past history of proven pelvic inflammatory disease does not establish the diagnosis at a later time. Laparoscopy can be very helpful in establishing the diagnosis of pelvic inflammatory disease, but, equally important, it can help eliminate the "stigma" of the diagnosis of chronic pelvic inflammatory disease from those who do not have it.[6]

In patients with chronic pelvic pain in whom the possibility of ovarian abnormalities, ovarian torsion, or chronic appendicitis is being considered, laparoscopy permits a much more thorough examination of the internal genitalia than a small appendectomy incision, while leaving open the possibility of corrective surgery during the same anesthetic if the condition warrants it.

In some patients adhesions of the tubes, uterus, or ovaries may be responsible for chronic or cyclic pain. These are usually due to prior surgical procedures and often can be lysed laparoscopically with relief of symptoms.[4]

Pelvic Mass

The discovery of a pelvic mass on physical examination in the postpubertal female, unlike her younger counterpart, does not always indicate the need for corrective surgery. A pregnancy test should always be obtained prior to invasive investigation. Laparoscopy will usually permit accurate definition and diagnosis of a pelvic mass. Some will require operation at the same time (ovarian torsion, tubal pregnancy), others can be treated under laparoscopic control (ovarian cysts), while still others require no operative treatment (salpingitis). Occasionally, no mass will be found, a lesser embarrassment after laparoscopy than after laparotomy!

Dysmenorrhea

Painful periods are often dismissed as "normal" or may be refractory to treatment with the usual analgesics or prostaglandin inhibitors. In these patients laparoscopy can be of value in establishing that there is no intrapelvic abnormality, or making the diagnosis when there is. Uterine anomalies are occasionally found, such as a unicornate uterus with obstruction of a dysplastic opposite horn with retained menstruum.[3] Similarly, cervical agenesis with uterine blockage can lead to pain. Endometriosis and chronic pelvic inflammatory disease are more common causes.

In well over half of adolescent girls with pelvic pain, laparoscopy will reveal the diagnosis without the requirement of laparotomy. Equally important, it can provide valuable information that there are no abnormalities of the internal genital organs.

References

1. Leape LL, Ramenofsky ML: Laparoscopy in children. Pediatrics 66:215–220, 1980
2. Cognat, M, Papathanassiou Z, Gomel V: Laparoscopy in infants and adolescents. J Reprod Med 13:11–12, 1974
3. Motashaw ND, Dastur A, Vaidya RA, et al: Laparoscopy for resolving Müllerian abnormalities. J Reprod Med 21:20–22, 1978
4. Goldstein D, deCholnoky C, Leventhal J, et al: New insights into the old problem of chronic pelvic pain. J Pediatr Surg 14:675–680, 1979
5. Kleppinger RK: Ovarian cyst fenestration via laparoscopy. J Reprod Med 21:16–19, 1978
6. Kleinhaus S, Hein K, Sheran M, et al: Laparoscopy for diagnosis and treatment of abdominal pain in adolescent girls. Arch Surg 112:1178–1179, 1977

Laparoscopy for Abdominal Pain

CHAPTER 14

Lucian L. Leape

Chronic Abdominal Pain

Few problems are as vexing for the pediatrician as the child with recurring or chronic abdominal pain. If there are other symptoms, such as vomiting, diarrhea, or urinary frequency, appropriate diagnostic studies will usually reveal the cause and lead to effective treatment. In a significant fraction of patients, particularly preadolescent girls, pain is the only symptom, and extensive laboratory and x-ray investigations are unrewarding. Laparoscopy can be of value in identifying the source of pain in some of these patients and is also helpful when negative in providing reassurance that certain other disease entities are not present.

Selection of Patients for Laparoscopy

Abdominal pain is usually not considered chronic until it has been present for a month or more. In addition to a complete history and physical examination, routine blood counts, urinalysis, urine culture, and selected x-ray and ultrasound examinations should be carried out before laparoscopy is contemplated. IVP and upper gastrointestinal series are most likely to be rewarding, although in the absence of specific symptoms other than pain, they are usually normal. Chronic constipation is a common cause of abdominal pain that must be ruled out by physical examination and specific treatment if necessary.

It is most important to identify the patient with psychogenic pain if possible. Specific clues must be adduced from the history to discover recent situational stress, and inquiries should be made regarding other possible psychosomatic symptoms. The diagnosis of psychogenic pain is not one of exclusion, but it can be difficult to establish if appropriate questioning is not carried out. In difficult but suspicious cases, the help of a child psychiatrist should be sought. In general, psychogenic abdominal pain tends to be poorly localized, seldom keeps the patient awake at night, and frequently disappears with admission to the hospital. Organ dysfunction pain, on the other hand, is more likely to be localized to one particular region of the abdomen and is no respecter of activity or sleep. If the patient exhibits reproducible localized tenderness on physical examination of the abdomen, laparoscopy is more likely to be rewarding.

Findings

In carefully selected patients, 40–50 percent of those undergoing laparoscopy for chronic or recurrent abdominal pain will be found to have a specific pathologic abnormality[1–3] (Table 14-1). If a surgically treatable lesion if found, such as an abnormal appendix, the operation can be carried out immediately following laparoscopy under the same anesthetic. Often patients will be found to have a pathologic condition that can be treated by means of the laparoscope or with ancillary instruments introduced through a separate cannula. Examples of this include removal of paraovarian cysts, fenestration of an ovarian cyst, lysis of adhesions (see Figure 37, p. vi), and removal of an accessory fallopian tube.

Nonsurgical causes of recurring or continuing abdominal pain, such as chronic salpingitis, regional enteritis, and perihepatitis, may be identified and appropriate drug therapy given. If the examination is completely negative, that information is of considerable value in reassuring the patient that there is no significant overlooked organic disease.

Table 14-1
Laparoscopic Findings in 46 Children with Chronic Abdominal Pain

Finding			
Negative		27	(59%)
Positive		19	(41%)
Chronic appendicitis	8		
Salpingitis	3		
Paraovarian cysts	2		
Ovarian cyst	1		
Accessory fallopian tube	1		
Regional enteritis	1		
Perihepatitis	1		
Omental adhesions	1		
Endometriosis	1		

If a pathologic condition is found at laparoscopy, its correction almost always leads to cure of the pain. If no abnormalities are noted, a small fraction of patients will nevertheless be improved following laparoscopy, presumably due to its placebo effect. Others may respond to psychotherapy. A significant fraction, however, will continue to have pain for months to years later.[1] Because of this, some have recommended that appendectomy be carried out if the examination is otherwise unremarkable, even if the appendix appears normal on laparoscopic examination. It has been demonstrated that some patients with chronic abdominal pain, particularly if localized to the right lower quadrant or the periumbilical region, will be cured by appendectomy. In these patients, appendiceal colic is thought to be due to fecal obstruction of the lumen.[4] Removal of an appendix that appears normal on laparoscopic examination may be indicated in patients with well-localized tenderness, but in those with generalized or diffuse pain it is unlikely to be helpful.

Pelvic Pain in Adolescent Females

Lower abdominal or pelvic pain is a common problem in postpubertal girls. Endometriosis as a cause of pelvic pain may be seen within the first year of menstruation[3] and is best diagnosed by laparoscopy. Ovarian and paraovarian cysts are not rare and can be treated laparoscopically in most cases. Adhesions from prior appendectomy or other operation may cause pain and can be lysed by the laparoscope.

The diagnosis of pelvic inflammatory disease may be established by laparoscopy. It has been demonstrated that a significant fraction of patients who were thought to have pelvic inflammatory disease or even a pelvic mass do not have it when laparoscopy is performed.[2] In these patients a negative laparoscopy is every bit as important as a positive one because it frees them from the stigma of the disease as well as the need to undergo useless antibiotic therapy.

Possible Appendicitis

The diagnosis of acute appendicitis, though frequently straightforward, often is not, and the physician is confronted with a patient who is clearly not well enough to return home but who also lacks clear-cut indications for operation. There may be localized pain and even some tenderness, but no evidence of guarding or other signs of peritoneal irritation, and the temperature and white blood count are normal. Most physicians recommend a period of in-hospital observation for the patients with equivocal findings, and if the symptoms disappear overnight no further treatment is indicated. If the patient worsens and develops peritoneal signs, then appendectomy is advised.

Laparoscopy can be of value in the patient with equivocal signs who does not show evidence of progressive disease typical of most patients with acute appendicitis. It is of particular value in children with complicating intercurrent disease, such as leukemia, steroid treatment for collagen disorders, or glomerulonephritis, or in patients with known regional enteritis. In such instances laparoscopy is preferable to watchful waiting, for if the patient does have appendicitis (see Figure 35, p. vi) it can be promptly corrected before complications occur in an already compromised host. Equally important, if the examination is negative (see Figure 34, p. vi), a high-risk patient is spared an unnecessary laparotomy. Laparoscopy has a distinct advantage over appendectomy if the patient does not have appendicitis, for it permits a better evaluation of other organs (such as ovaries and tubes) than is usually possible through a standard appendectomy incision.

The diagnosis of appendicitis is made at laparoscopy if the appendix is seen to be inflamed, is covered by adherent omentum, or is surrounded by an inflammatory exudate. If the appendix cannot be visualized, two possibilities exist: that it is bound down by inflammatory adhesions, or that its natural anatomic position is retrocecal and therefore not accessible to examination. It is better to remove the appendix that cannot be visualized by laparoscopy than to assume it is merely retrocecal and uninflamed. Indeed, the retrocecal position may well be the reason why the findings are equivocal.

It is essential that the appendix be completely examined—from tip to base—before the decision is made that appendicitis is not present. Localized or segmental involvement can exist and be missed if the examination is not complete.

Results of laparoscopy for highly selected patients with equivocal signs of appendicitis reveal that about 50 percent of these patients will indeed have appendicitis[5] (Table 14-2). Appendectomy should be carried out at the same time. A significant fraction of patients will be found to have no abnormalities, and these will be spared an unnecessary operation. The remaining patients often can be treated nonoperatively, although other conditions (such as ovarian torsion, Meckel's diverticulitis, tumor abscess, and so forth) may require surgical treatment.

Judicious application of laparoscopy to patients with equivocal findings of appendicitis significantly reduces the negative appendectomy rate.[5] This does not mean, however, that laparoscopy should be used in patients with definite evidence of appendicitis. These patients require an operation. In practice only about 10–20 percent of patients with questionable appendicitis will require laparoscopy.

The use of laparoscopy in patients with possible appendicitis has been criticized on two accounts: the patient is subjected to a general anesthetic without the benefit of an appendectomy (for which he may later return), and it may be impossible to tell for sure that appendicitis does not exist by examining the outside of the appen-

Table 14-2
Laparoscopic Findings in 42 Children with Suspected Appendicitis

Finding		Number	Percent
Acute appendicitis		23	(55%)
Normal		9 *	(21%)
Other		10	(24%)
Leukemic infiltrates	2*		
Mittleschmerz	2		
Salpingitis	2		
Torsion paraovarian cyst	1		
Ruptured ovarian cyst	1		
Tumor abscess	1		
Crohn's disease	1		

*One patient in each of these groups later proved to have appendicitis.

dix through the laparoscope. Every surgeon has removed an appendix he thought was grossly normal only to have the pathologist tell him later that it was inflamed. Nevertheless, these theoretical considerations are countered by the experience of finding a variety of other conditions that might have been overlooked if a standard appendectomy were performed. The great advantage of laparoscopy is that it permits a much more thorough examination of the pelvis than does laparotomy unless a large incision is used.

References

1. Leape LL, Ramenofsky ML: Laparoscopy in children. Pediatrics 66:215–220, 1980
2. Kleinhaus S, Hein K, Sheran M, et al: Laparoscopy for diagnosis and treatment of abdominal pain in adolescent girls. Arch 112:1178–1179, 1977
3. Goldstein D, deCholnoky C, Leventhal J, et al: New insights into the old problem of chronic pelvic pain. J Pediatr Surg 14:675–680, 1979
4. Schisgall RM: Appendiceal colic in childhood. The role of inspissated casts of stool within the appendix. Ann Surg 192:687–693, 1980
5. Leape LL, Ramenofsky ML: Laparoscopy for questionable appendicitis: can it reduce the negative appendectomy rate? Ann Surg 191:410–413, 1980

Laparoscopy in the Diagnosis and Treatment of Malfunctioning Ventriculoperitoneal Shunts

CHAPTER 15

Bradley M. Rodgers
John K. Vries
James L. Talbert

Originally described by Kausch in 1905,[1] the ventriculoperitoneal shunt has become the most widely employed technique for the treatment of hydrocephalus. Nevertheless, this procedure has been associated with a significant incidence of intra-abdominal complications.[2] The most common of these have included peritonitis, visceral perforation, volvulus, cerebrospinal fluid (CSF) ascites, and inguinal hernia. Grosfeld et al. reported these complications to have occurred with a frequency as high as 25

Based on Rodgers BM, Vries JK, Talbert JL: Laparoscopy in the diagnosis and treatment of malfunctioning ventriculoperitoneal shunts in children. J Pediatr Surg 13:247–253, 1978. Reprinted by permission.

percent.[3] A further complication leading to failure of the shunt system has been encystation of the peritoneal end of the catheter. In most of the cases of this latter problem, definitive diagnosis has required exploratory laparotomy, and treatment has usually necessitated removal of the peritoneal catheter and conversion to an entirely different shunt system.[4]

Over the past several years, important advances in rod lens optical systems have permitted the manufacture of miniaturized endoscopic equipment (see Chapter 12). These instruments have made possible the performance of laparoscopy in small infants and children with comparative ease and safety.[5] The present report describes the use of laparoscopy in the diagnosis and treatment of encystation of the abdominal limb of ventriculoperitoneal shunt systems.

Materials and Methods

Laparoscopy was performed in 4 hydrocephalic children with malfunctioning ventriculoperitoneal shunts. The shunt used in each case was the Hakim system with a medium pressure valve. In each case the site of the malfunction was suspected to be the abdominal catheter because of difficulty compressing the pumping chamber or the presence of fluid dissecting along the distal portion of the shunt track.

In all infants laparoscopy was performed under general anesthesia to allow controlled ventilation. Under sterile conditions, the Veress pneumoperitoneum needle (Karl Storz No. 26120J) was inserted through the lower midline and the abdominal cavity was insufflated with carbon dioxide to a pressure of 30 cm H_2O. In procedures requiring a long operative time and repeated carbon dioxide insufflation, we have noted a mild elevation of arterial PCO_2 in these small infants, with a resultant compensatory tachypnea. Controlled ventilation is useful in these situations. The needle was then removed, and the pediatric laparoscopic trocar and cannula (Karl Storz No. 26181H) was inserted into the anterior abdominal cavity through the same infraumbilical midline track. Using the Hopkins forward-viewing telescope (Karl Storz No. 27018A), we obtained an excellent view of the entire anterior abdominal cavity, upper abdominal viscera, and pelvis. The tip of the peritoneal catheter was located by following the catheter from its point of insertion through the abdominal wall. A second pediatric laparoscopic trocar and cannula were then inserted adjacent to the first, and the biopsy forceps (Karl Storz No. 26180F) was inserted through this cannula. The end of the catheter was freed from surrounding adhesions or encystation and moved to a point in the abdominal cavity determined to be free of adhesions. The carbon dioxide remaining within the abdominal cavity was evacuated, both cannulas were removed, and the puncture wounds sutured closed.

Case Reports

Case 1: R.M.

This 1540-gm male infant developed hydrocephalus secondary to an intraventricular hemorrhage shortly following birth. Control of this condition necessitated insertion of a ventriculoperitoneal shunt at 2 weeks of age. Seven weeks following placement of the shunt, the valve eroded through the skin of the scalp and the infant developed *Candida* ventriculitis. Management of this infection required removal of the ventriculoperitoneal shunt and use of external ventricular drainage with instillation of intrathecal antibiotics. A second ventriculoperitoneal shunt was subsequently inserted. Three months later, the patient was readmitted to the hospital with an inappropriately increasing head circumference associated with vomiting. CSF cultures revealed recurrent *Candida* ventriculitis with the organism sensitive to 5-fluorocytosine. The shunt system was replaced and the patient was treated for 3 months with this antibiotic. At the conclusion of the course of therapy, the patient was readmitted to the hospital with fluid dissecting along the shunt track and difficulty in depressing the shunt chamber. Abdominal radiographs revealed fixation of the catheter tip within a cystic mass in the midabdomen (Figure 15-1A, B). Laparoscopy was performed and a large right-upper-quadrant cyst was encountered. The wall of the cyst was punctured with the biopsy forceps, and multiple fragments of the wall were removed. Although the catheter was easily visualized, it was not thought necessary to remove it from the decompressed cyst. Following this procedure, the shunt functioned normally until the patient was readmitted 8 months later with increasing irritability and a palpable abdominal mass. Sonography demontrated a recurrent cyst located anteriorly within the peritoneal cavity. Laparoscopy at that time identified the catheter within a large recurrent anterior abdominal cyst. A portion of the wall was removed from the cyst, and the catheter was moved into the left pelvis. Cultures of peritoneal fluid at this time revealed *Candida* organisms. Ten days later, the patient was readmitted to the hospital with fever and irritability. On this admission an exploratory laparotomy was performed and the wall of a large anterior abdominal cyst was excised. Cultures of the fluid within this cyst again grew *Candida* species and the patient was treated with 5-fluorocytosine. Fever persisted and was accompanied by increasing abdominal girth. The entire ventriculoperitoneal shunt system was removed, to be replaced 2 weeks later with a ventriculopleural shunt. The patient remained asymptomatic with a normally functioning shunt system for 26 months and has subsequently been lost to followup.

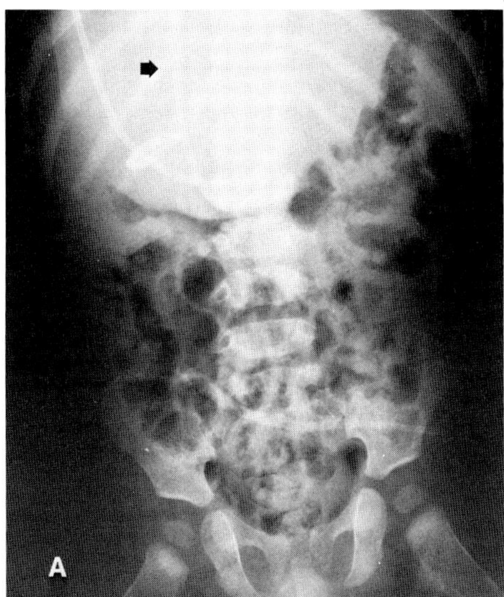

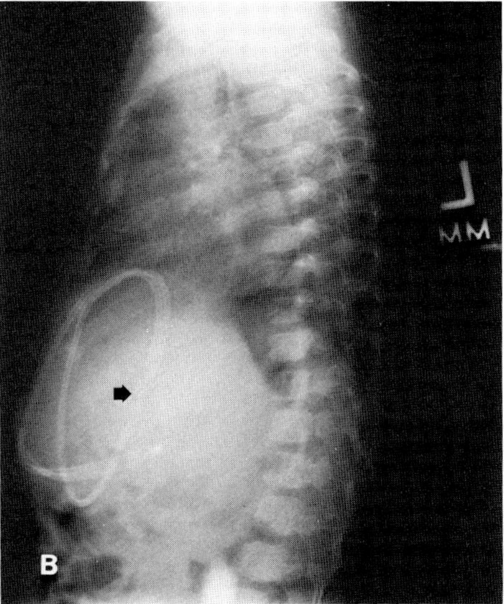

Figure 15-1. *Case 1: Supine (A) and lateral (B) abdominal radiographs showing the tip of the peritoneal catheter (arrows) to be within a soft-tissue density in the right upper quadrant. The transverse colon is displaced caudad, indicating a space-occupying lesion in this region. Sonography confirmed the presence of a cyst in the right upper quadrant. (From Rodgers BM, Vries JK, Talbert JL: Laparoscopy in the diagnosis and treatment of malfunctioning ventriculoperitoneal shunts in children. J Pediatr Surg 13:247–253, 1978. With permission.)*

Case 2: C.L.

This 4200-gm female infant was noted at birth to have congenital hydrocephalus that was confirmed by EMI scan (computerized transaxial tomography). A ventriculoperitoneal shunt system was inserted on the third day of life. She was readmitted to the hospital 2 months later with skin erosion over the shunt reservoir. Cultures of the CSF grew *Staphylococcus epidermidis* and the shunt system was removed and external ventriculostomy drainage established. After 10 days of intensive antibiotic therapy, a second ventriculoperitoneal shunt was placed. Five weeks later the patient was readmitted to the hospital with an inappropriately increasing head circumference. Abdominal radiographs revealed fixation of the catheter tip in the left upper quadrant (Figure 15-2A) and sonography showed a small cystic accumulation in this area (Figure 15-2B). At laparoscopy the tip of the peritoneal shunt was found in the left upper quadrant within a fluid-filled cyst surrounded by omentum (Figure 15-3). The cyst was punctured with the biopsy instrument and the shunt catheter was removed from this area and transferred to the right upper quadrant. Cultures of the cyst fluid were negative. Three weeks following discharge she was readmitted to the hospital with lethargy and increasing head size and was noted to have fluid dissecting along the shunt track. Laparoscopy was repeated and the catheter tip was found to be entangled within omentum and the gastrohepatic ligament in the right upper quadrant. The catheter was removed from this area and placed in the lower abdomen. This patient was asymptomatic with a properly functioning shunt system 24 months later.

Case 3: B.W.

This full-term male infant was born with a thoracic meningomyelocele that was repaired during the first day of life. He subsequently developed hydrocephalus and underwent ventriculoperitoneal shunting at 3 months of age. Two months later he was admitted to the hospital for repair of a large ventral hernia and at that time was noted to have fluid dissecting along the shunt track. He was taken to surgery for repair of his ventral hernia, and the peritoneal end of the shunt was explored and replaced within the peritoneal cavity, without

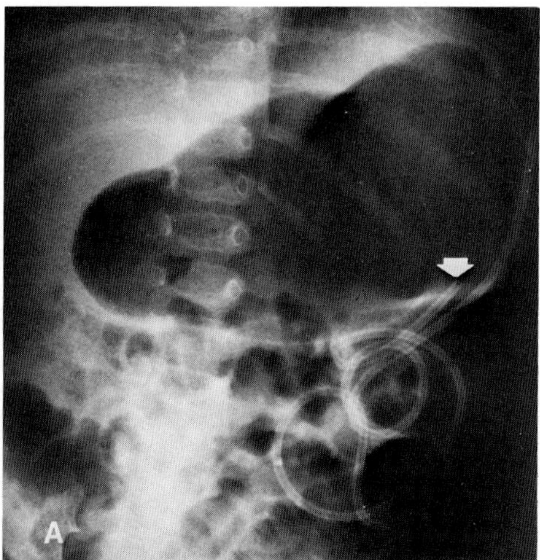

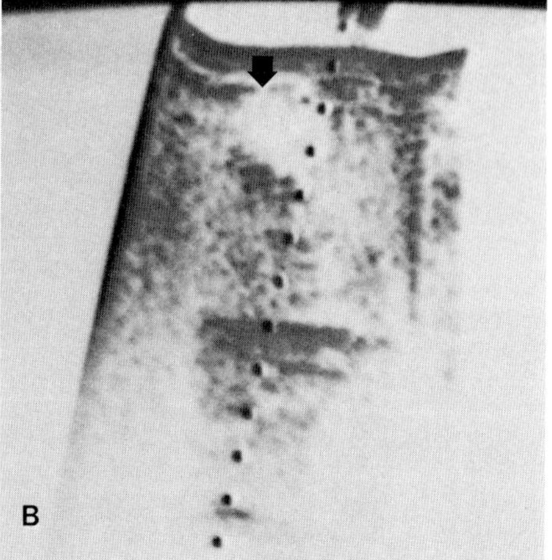

Figure 15-2. *Case 2: (A) Supine abdominal radiograph demonstrating the tip of the peritoneal catheter (arrow) to lie within the left upper quadrant. This tip remained stationary on multiple abdominal radiographs. (B) Sonography in the sagittal plane of the left upper quadrant confirms a small cystic lesion (arrow) lying anteriorly in this region. (From Rodgers BM, Vries JK, Talbert JL: Laparoscopy in the diagnosis and treatment of malfunctioning ventriculoperitoneal shunts in children. J Pediatr Surg 13:247–253, 1978. With permission.)*

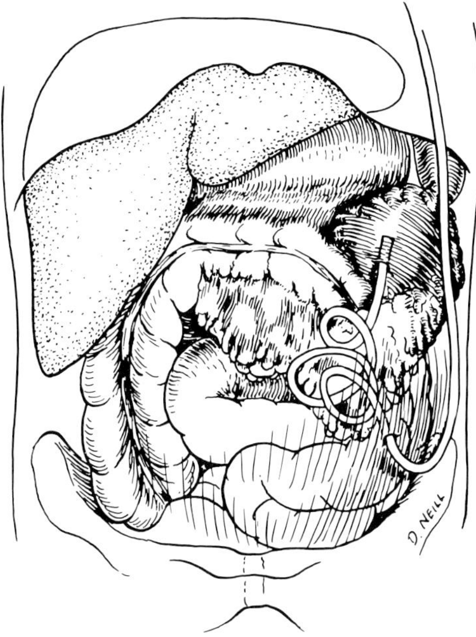

Figure 15-3. *Case 2: Illustration of peritoneal catheter entering a 6-cm pseudocyst surrounded by omentum. The pseudocyst impinged inferiorly on the splenic flexure of the colon and superiorly on the spleen and stomach. (From Rodgers BM, Vries JK, Talbert JL: Laparoscopy in the diagnosis and treatment of malfunctioning ventriculoperitoneal shunts in children. J Pediatr Surg 13:247–253, 1978. With permission.)*

definitive findings. He underwent posterior spinal fusion 2 months later for kyphosis at which time the shunt appeared to be functioning normally. Four months after initial shunt revision, he was readmitted to the hospital with an inappropriately increasing head circumference and difficulty in compressing his shunt pump. He was also noted to have bilateral inguinal hernias. Abdominal radiographs obtained in multiple positions demonstrated fixation of the catheter tip in the right lower quadrant (Figure 15-4A) and ultrasonic examination demonstrated a cystic mass surrounding the shunt tip. The patient underwent bilateral herniorrhaphy. During the course of this procedure, laparoscopy was performed by passing the laparoscopic telescope through the right hernia sac and the biopsy forceps through the left hernia sac (Figure 15-4B). Pursestring sutures were used about the base of the hernia sacs in order to allow effective carbon dioxide insufflation into the abdominal cavity. The end of the shunt was identified and found to be entrapped by omentum in the right lower quadrant. The forceps were used to dissect the shunt free, and the tip of the catheter was grasped and moved to a new abdominal location in an area free of adhesions. Cultures of the peritoneal fluid were negative. Thirty-eight months postoperatively, the patient was asymptomatic with a properly functioning shunt system.

Case 4: P.E.

This full-term female infant was born with a lumbar meningomyelocele that was repaired during the first day of life. At 2 weeks of age she developed hydrocephalus that was treated with a ventriculoperitoneal shunt. At 3 months of age she was admitted to the hospital because of fluid dissecting along the course of her shunt catheter and difficulty in compressing the shunt pump. Abdominal radiographs in multiple views showed fixation of the peritoneal end of the shunt in the midabdomen (Figure 15-5). However, no cystic lesion could be identified by sonography. Laparoscopy was performed and the tip of the catheter was found to be entrapped within the falciform ligament and surrounded by omentum. The shunt was easily removed from its entrapment with the biopsy forceps and replaced in the lower abdomen. Cultures of the peritoneal fluid were negative. This patient's hydrocephalus was under satisfactory control with a properly functioning shunt system 29 months postoperatively.

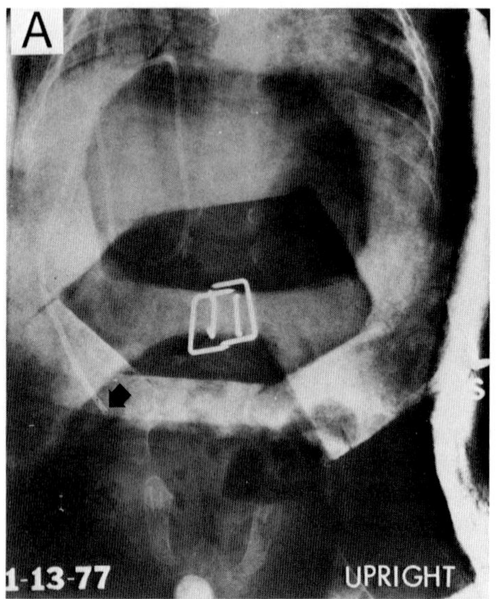

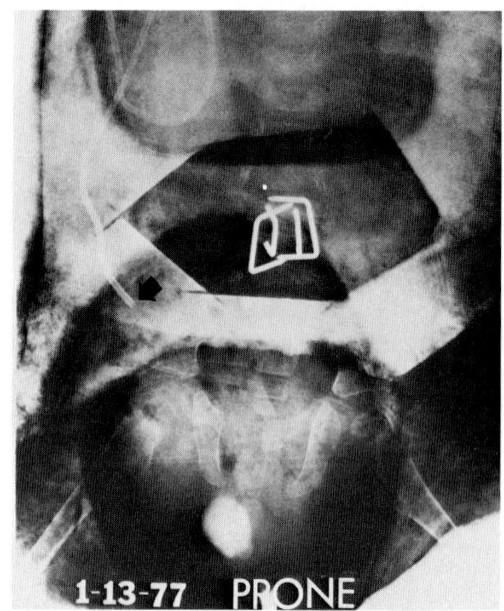

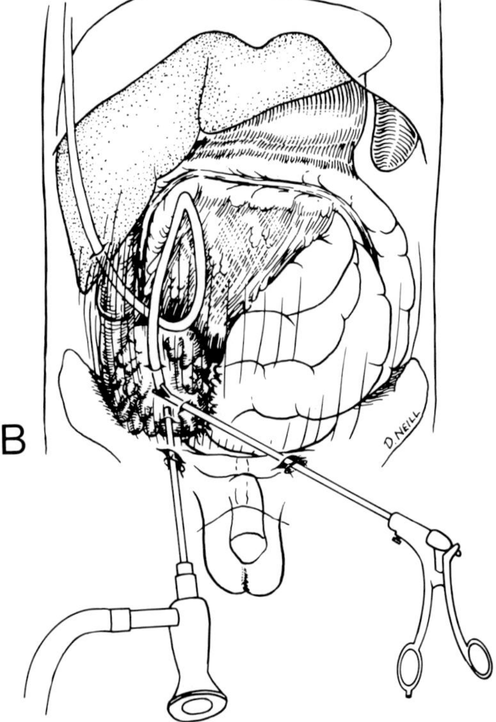

Figure 15-4. *Case 3: (A) Upright and prone abdominal radiographs demonstrating the tip of the peritoneal catheter (arrows) to be fixed in position in the right lower quadrant. (B) Laparoscopy was performed through bilateral inguinal hernia sacs and a 5-cm pseudocyst was observed. The pseudocyst was covered with omentum and lay anterior to the cecum. The catheter was removed from this area and placed within the left lower quadrant. (From Rodgers BM, Vries JK, Talbert JL: Laparoscopy in the diagnosis and treatment of malfunctioning ventriculoperitoneal shunts in children. J Pediatr Surg 13:247–253, 1978. With permission.)*

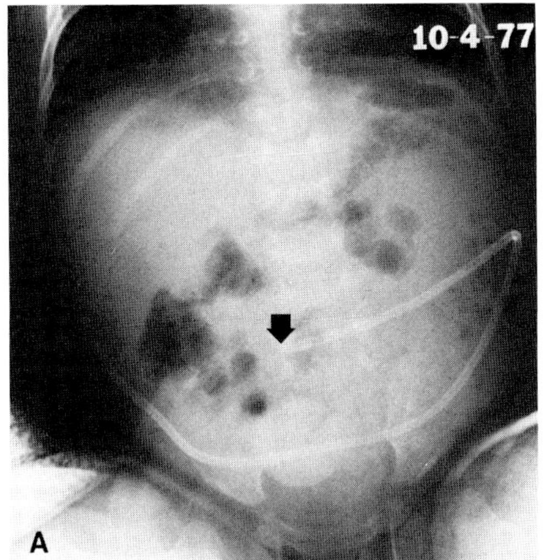

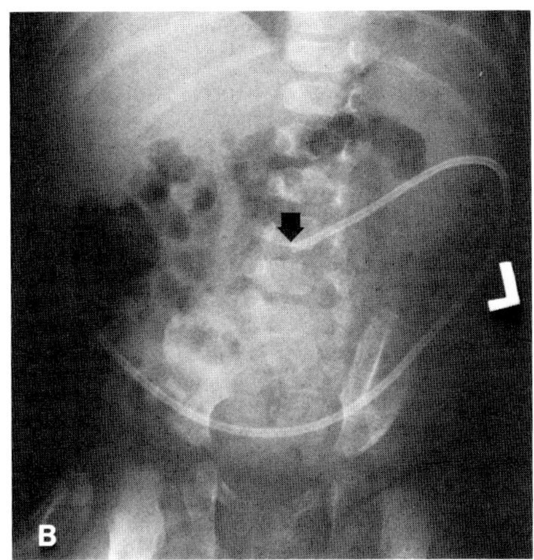

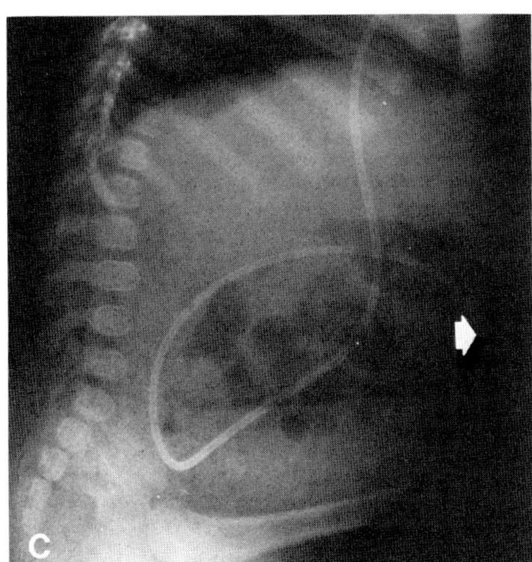

Figure 15-5. *Case 4: (A) Upright, (B) prone, and (C) lateral abdominal radiographs demonstrate fixation of the peritoneal limb of the catheter (arrows) anteriorly in the region of the falciform ligament. (From Rodgers BM, Vries JK, Talbert JL: Laparoscopy in the diagnosis and treatment of malfunctioning ventriculoperitoneal shunts in children. J Pediatr Surg 13:247–253, 1978. With permission.)*

Discussion

Although the long-term results with ventriculoperitoneal shunt systems have usually been quite satisfactory, significant numbers of abdominal complications have been reported in all series. The most common abdominal complication noted has been the development of inguinal hernias, which occurs in approximately 17 percent of these children.[3] Less common but considerably more serious complications include visceral perforation by the peritoneal catheter, volvulus about the catheter with intestinal obstruction, and the development of cerebrospinal fluid cysts around the end of the peritoneal catheter. This last complication has been recognized with increasing frequency since its initial description by Jackson in 1955.[6] The most important clinical signs indicating malfunction of the peritoneal limb of a ventriculoperitoneal shunt are (1) inappropriately increasing head circumference, with or without associated neurologic signs, such as lethargy and vomiting; (2) resistance to depression of the shunt pump; and (3) dissection of fluid along the shunt track, beginning at either the abdominal or ventral end. Rarely have these intraperitoneal pseudocysts been palpable on physical examination. Abdominal radiographs have, on occasion, been useful in identifying the pseudocysts, and injections of radiopaque material[3] or radionuclides[7] into the shunt system have reportedly diagnosed the complication. In our experience, abdominal radiographs taken in multiple positions have demonstrated the end of the ventriculoperitoneal catheter to be fixed in position within the abdomen in every patient with abdominal entrapment or encystation. In contrast, children with normally functioning ventriculoperitoneal shunt systems demonstrate free movement of the peritoneal catheter within the abdominal cavity on change of position. In patients with abnormal abdominal radiographs, sonography of the peritoneal cavity in the region of the tip of the peritoneal catheter has been used to confirm the diagnosis of encystation. A cyst may not be evident, however, in the presence of entrapment of the catheter tip, as in our Case 4.

The process of encystation begins with entrapment of the tip of the peritoneal catheter within one of the peritoneal reflections or omentum with subsequent obstruction to free flow of the cerebrospinal fluid. Entrapment of the catheter tip alone may be sufficient to increase resistance to flow and cause symptoms; or persistent entrapment may progress to pseudocyst formation and development of symptoms and physical findings of an abdominal mass. Reviewing our experience and that of others, there appears to be two factors that may increase the liklihood of encystation of the peritoneal limb of the catheter: (1) the presence of adhesions from previous operative procedures or infected peritoneal fluid, which appears to significantly enhance the possibility of entrapment; and (2) placement of the catheter tip in the upper abdomen in the region of the omentum and gastrohepatic, gastrocolonic, and falciform ligaments, which may entrap the catheter tip.

Previous reports describing encystation of the peritoneal limb of this shunt system have recommended laparotomy and complete removal of the peritoneal catheter with conversion to a new shunt system as the most satisfactory mode of management.[4] We believe that laparoscopy offers several advantages over this method of therapy: (1) By the use of laparoscopy, it is possibie to visualize the peritoneal catheter in situ and make a precise diagnosis of the cause of malfunction of the shunt system; (2) peritoneal fluid and tissue can be easily obtained for culture during laparoscopy; (3) the entire abdominal cavity can be visualized and a region most suitable for positioning of the shunt catheter may be determined; and (4) the use of laparoscopy rather than repeated laparotomy avoids formation of new adhesions within the abdominal cavity and should therefore reduce the likelihood of recurrent entrapment.

Three of our 4 patients currently have normally functioning peritoneal shunt systems, despite the need for a second laparoscopic relocation in one of them (Case 2). The infant with chronic *Candida* ventriculitis and peritonitis (Case 1) suffered continued encystation despite two laparoscopic repositionings. Failure of this technique can be expected in the presence of active peritonitis, and this child's shunt was ultimately converted to a ventriculopleural system. This experience suggests to us that it is possible to salvage many malfunctioning ventriculoperitoneal shunt systems by retrieval of the tip of the peritoneal catheter from within a pseudocyst or omental entrapment using pediatric laparoscopic equipment. The technique of laparoscopic repositioning of malfunctioning ventriculoperitoneal shunts has proven rapid and easy to perform, and there have been no operative complications. Morgan has reported similar success in repositioning the peritoneal catheter entrapped by abdominal adhesions.[8] In addition, Morgan has employed laparoscopy on four occasions to retrieve shunt catheters that have come loose within the peritoneal cavity, a complication we have not encountered. Close surveillance of children with ventriculoperitoneal shunts, including the use of abdominal radiographs in multiple positions and selective use of sonography, may allow earlier diagnosis of catheter entrapment and more successful treatment.

References

1. Kausch W, cited by Haynes IS: Congenital internal hydrocephalus: its treatment by drainage of the cisterna magna into the cranial sinuses. Ann Surg 57:449–484, 1913
2. Davidson RI: Peritoneal bypass in the treatment of hydrocephalus: historical review and abdominal complications. J Neurol Neurosurg Psychiatry 39:640–646, 1976
3. Grosfeld JL, Cooney DR, Smith J, et al: Intra-abdominal complications following ventriculoperitoneal shunt procedures. Pediatrics 54:791–796, 1974
4. Fischer EG, Schillito J: Large abdominal cysts: a complication of peritoneal shunts. Report of three cases. J Neurosurg 31:441–444, 1969
5. Gans SL, Berci G: Peritoneoscopy in infants and children. J Pediatr Surg 8:399–405, 1973
6. Jackson IJ, Snodgrass SR: Peritoneal shunts in the treatment of hydrocephalus and increased intracranial pressure: a 4-year survey of 62 patients. J Neurosurg 12:216–222, 1955
7. Di Chiro G, Grove AS: Evaluation of surgical and spontaneous cerebrospinal fluid shunts by isotope scanning. J Neurosurg 24:743–748, 1966
8. Morgan WW: The use of peritoneoscopy in the diagnosis and treatment of complications of ventriculoperitoneal shunts in children. J Pediatr Surg 14:180–181, 1979

Laparoscopy for Trauma

CHAPTER 16

Edward Austin
Stephen L. Gans

In the infant and childhood age groups the incidence of trauma-related injuries and death is of major significance. In an effort to minimize any unnecessary operative procedures, and to decrease patient morbidity, we started investigating the use of advanced optical equipment in 1977 and presented a preliminary report of our results in 1980.[1] We are now able to recommend this method as a rapid, accurate, and safe assessment of intra-abdominal injuries.

A common method of diagnosing intra-abdominal injuries has been the sampling of peritoneal fluid by abdominal tap or peritoneal lavage to detect the presence of blood, white blood cells, intestinal contents, or pancreatic enzymes. Many institutions adhere to the belief that the presence of bloody fluid in the peritoneal cavity following blunt trauma is an indication for immediate laparotomy. However, this practice results in a high incidence of unwarranted laparotomy. The absence of blood is generally accepted as being unreliable and, in such situations, other criteria must be employed to arrive at a decision for or against exploration. Nevertheless, the widespread use of peritoneal lavage has reduced the incidence of missed intra-abdominal injuries and has resulted in reduced morbidity and mortality from blunt abdominal trauma. It is important to note, however, that the presence of blood in the peritoneal cavity indicates only that bleeding has taken place, and is not necessarily continuing, and that peritoneal lavage does not identify the origin of the bleeding. There are a number of injuries that may result in hemoperitoneum but do not require surgical intervention. Two such situations are pelvic fractures and retroperitoneal hematomas, which frequently give false-positive lavage interpretations and result in unnecessary and nonproductive laparotomies. Furthermore, the nonoperative approach to the stable child with a splenic injury is one that has gained considerable acceptance by pediatric surgeons. Obviously, an unnecessary laparotomy on a seriously injured child should be avoided whenever possible because it delays other important diagnostic and therapeutic procedures and results in undue morbidity and sometimes mortality. We therefore advocate, *when indicated,* direct visualization of the intra-abdominal viscera by means of emergency laparoscopy performed as soon as possible following arrival of the patient at the hospital.

Indications

An infant or child with severe *multiple organ system trauma,* resulting most frequently from a motor vehicle collision, is one that requires the most expedient diagnosis of internal injuries and prompt therapeutic intervention (see Table 16-1). A child with significant head, chest, and extremity trauma should always raise the suspicion of a serious intra-abdominal injury. Laparoscopic observation of the intra-abdominal viscera will rule in or out a life-threatening injury and allow the workup and treatment to proceed in an appropriate manner. Before sending the child for a head scan, multiple orthopedic x-rays, or other prolonged procedures, the physician can feel confident that the child will not exsanguinate from an unrecognized intra-abdominal catastrophe.

Physical examination of an *unconscious* child is extremely difficult and fraught with uncertainty due to the urgency of the situation. Lacking appropriate signs of tenderness, rigidity, and guarding, the diagnosis of an abdominal injury in an unconscious patient may be expedited by emergency laparoscopy.

Laboratory findings of an *unexplained low or falling hemoglobin,* elevated liver or pancreatic enzymes, and hematuria indicate the need for further investigation of the intra-abdominal viscera. The liver and spleen are the most frequently injured abdominal organs and may be adequately studied by radioisotope and computerized scanning techniques. These methods are, however, time-consuming and may require moving the patient to other areas of the hospital. They also do not indicate whether the injury is responsible for acute bleeding or whether the bleeding has stopped. These non-invasive studies are more appropriate for stable patients without other serious injuries, in whom time is not a critical factor.

Table 16-1
Indications for Emergency Laparoscopy

Multiple organ system trauma
Impaired sensorium
Unexplained falling hemoglobin
Equivocal abdominal examination
Stab wound with questionable abdominal wall penetration

A patient who has undergone serial *equivocal abdominal examinations* and whose findings are sufficient to elicit a high index of suspicion in the surgeon's mind may be a candidate for laparoscopy. In these situations, laparoscopy may provide the only alternative to laparotomy and may substantially reduce the number of negative explorations of such patients.

In patients with *stab wounds with questionable penetration of the abdominal cavity,* laparoscopy may be used to observe the undersurface of the abdominal wall and document whether it has actually been perforated.

Method

Laparoscopy, either electively or emergently, is best performed in the operating room. However, in certain instances in unstable patients, it can be safely performed in the emergency room or intensive care unit, using local anesthesia. The entire instrument set, including the light source, may be quickly and easily moved anywhere for immediate use. The procedure may be completed in 15 minutes by an experienced laparoscopist with a nurse assisting.

The emergency laparoscopy set is shown in Figure 16-1. While the assistant is preparing the skin of the abdomen with a suitable antiseptic solution, the instrument tray is opened and checked. Sterile drapes are placed, leaving the entire abdominal wall exposed. A local anesthetic (Xylocaine 0.5 percent), is injected just below the umbilicus in the midline. A 3 mm stab wound is made with a scalpel and bluntly spread down to the midline fascia with a small hemostat. The skin is tented upward and the single-puncture needle-cannula (see Figure 11-6A) is advanced through the fascia into the peritoneal cavity. A noticeable snap is felt and heard as the blunt stylet springs forward upon entering the abdominal cavity. Five cc of saline is injected and then aspirated to confirm that the bowel has not been entered. A small amount of air is insufflated with a rubber bulb connected to the cannula. The needle component is removed from the cannula and replaced by the telescope (see Figure 11-6B). The area underlying the puncture site should be examined first, to confirm that no injury has been produced by introduction of the instruments. The abdomen is *gradually* insufflated with air while a systematic examination of all quadrants of the abdomen is carried out. The assistant should be carefully observing the patient for impairment of respiration or other signs of instability.

Results

When there are no positive findings, the procedure is quickly terminated and other surgical or diagnostic procedures may be resumed. Prolonged laparoscopic examination, as might be required for assessing a tumor or congenital anomaly, is not appropriate in the traumatized child. Positive findings should be easily recognized by an experienced laparoscopist and their significance correctly appreciated. Bile or food particles indicate a ruptured stomach or intestine and immediate laparotomy is mandated. Blood is easily recognized, but the quantity and source should be determined. Placement of a second cannula is frequently useful in this regard. It may be

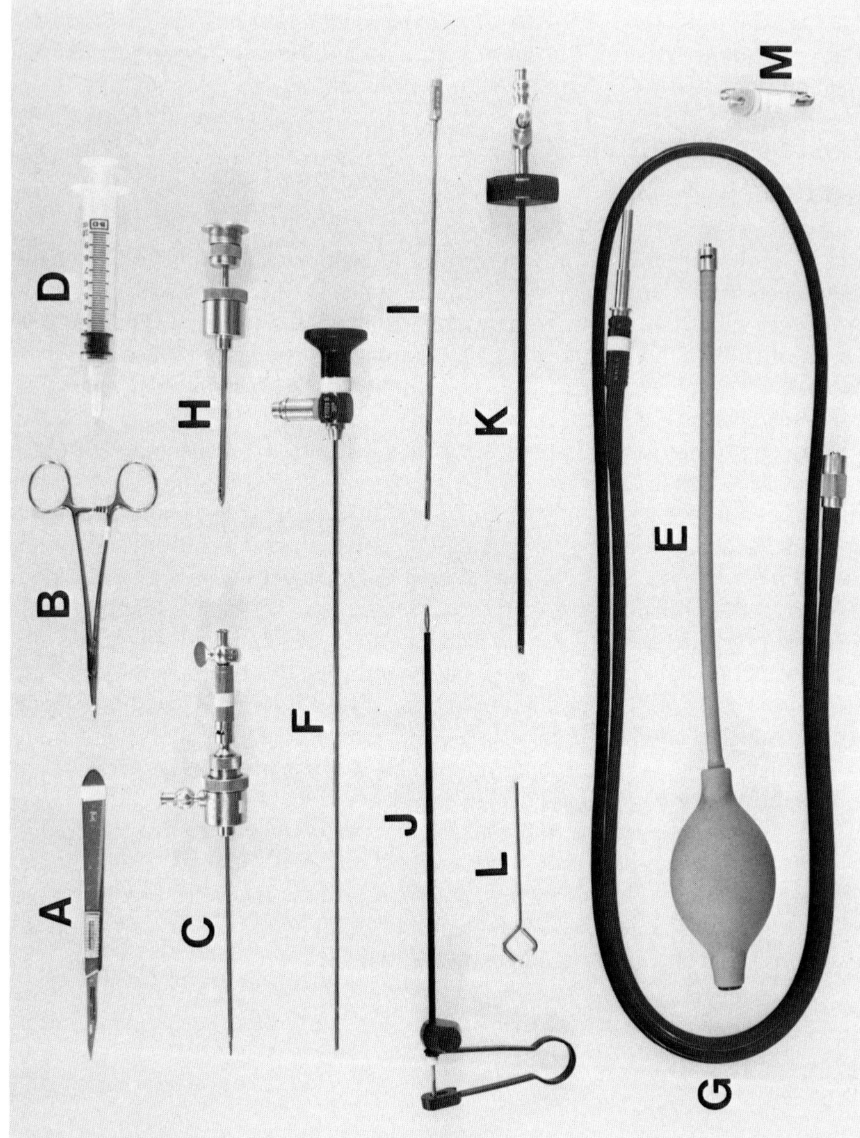

Figure 16-1. *Sterile instrument set for emergency pediatric laparoscopy. See Table 16-2.*

Table 16-2
Equipment for Pediatric Emergency Laparoscopy: Sterile Setup (See Figure 16-1)

For Examination	
A.	Pointed knife, No. 11 blade
B.	Mosquito hemostats, straight and curved
C.	Gans-Austin single puncture combined Veress needle and examining cannula
D.	Syringe, 10 ml, and normal saline, 50 ml
E.	Insufflation bulb
F.	Hopkins forward-oblique telescope, 30°
G.	Fiberoptic light cable
*	Teaching attachment
For Further Manipulation or Instrumentation	
H.	Trochar and cannula, O.D. 4 mm, for manipulating instruments
I.	Palpation probe
J.	Grasping forceps
K.	Suction-coagulation cannula probe
*	Cable to connect above to electrosurgical unit
L.	Desufflation key
M.	Spare parts (gaskets, washers)
*	Sponges, skin suture, needle holder, and scissors

*Not shown in Figure 16-1.

safely placed in any area of the abdominal cavity, as dictated by the initial findings, under direct vision through the telescope. Several useful maneuvers can be performed through the second cannula. A suction catheter can be inserted to remove any blood that is present and permit clear observation of a bleeding site as well as quantify the rapidity of hemorrhage (see Figure 38, p. vi). The observer may find that bleeding from a minor splenic or hepatic tear has slowed or stopped completely (see Figures 39 and 40, p. vi). This is frequently the case with small liver capsular tears at the insertion of the falciform ligament, which rarely require surgical repair. The suction catheter can also be used to obtain samples of peritoneal fluid for amylase and WBC analysis. An atraumatic grasping forceps or palpation probe may be inserted through the secondary cannula to maneuver omentum and bowel loops for better observation.

After laparoscopy is completed, the air is allowed to escape through the cannula by inserting a key to open the one-way valve. The cannula is then removed and the puncture sites are closed with sutures or clips and small dressings are placed. The trauma team may then proceed with further workup confident that an intra-abdominal injury has not been overlooked.

Contraindications

Laparoscopy is not a substitute for immediate laparotomy in a child with an obvious surgical abdomen and should not delay immediate preparation for surgery.

Other general contraindications for laparoscopy, including multiple previous surgeries, abdominal distention, and peritonitis, pertain to the traumatized child as well.

References

1. Austin E, Gans SL: Emergency laparoscopy in infants and children. Presented at the Thirteenth Annual Meeting of the Pacific Association of Pediatric Surgeons, Colorado Springs, Colo, May 21–24, 1980

Index

Page numbers followed by *t* indicate tables. Page numbers in italics indicate figures.

a
b
3 c
4 d
5 e
6 f
7 g
8 h
9 i
80 j